Institutional abuse

Public inquiries, court cases and Government statements concerning institutional abuse in different settings have generated considerable interest in this topic, and have highlighted the need for the caring professions to develop preventive strategies and appropriate responses to this form of abuse.

Institutional Abuse brings together a number of different accounts of institutional abuse from leading academics and researchers. Using a life course perspective, four areas are covered: the institutional abuse of children, of adults with learning disabilities, of adults with mental health problems and of older people. Each section includes a critical overview, analysis of current research and a chapter reporting on users' experiences of abuse. This book aims to develop our understanding of how institutional abuse can be prevented and survivors' needs can be meet.

Institutional Abuse will be of interest to those studying social work and social policy, practitioners and managers, researchers and policy makers.

Nicky Stanley, **Jill Manthorpe** and **Bridget Penhale** are lecturers based in the School of Community and Health Studies at the University of Hull.

Institutional abuse

Perspectives across the life course

Edited by Nicky Stanley, Jill Manthorpe and Bridget Penhale

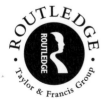

London and New York

First published 1999
by Routledge
11 New Fetter Lane, London EC4P 4EE

Simultaneously published in the USA and Canada
by Routledge
29 West 35th Street, New York, NY 10001

Routledge is an imprint of the Taylor & Francis Group

© 1999 selection and editorial matter, Nicky Stanley, Jill Manthorpe
and Bridget Penhale; individual chapters, the contributors

Typeset in Times by Routledge
Printed and bound in Great Britain by TJ International Ltd, Padstow, Cornwall

British Library Cataloguing in Publication Data
A catalogue record for this book is available from the British Library

Library of Congress Cataloguing in Publication Data
Institutional abuse : perspectives across the life course / edited by
Nicky Stanley, Jill Manthorpe and Bridget Penhale.
    p. cm.
Includes bibliographical references.
1. Institutional care–Great Britain. 2. Children–Institutional
care–Great Britain. 3. Child abuse–Great Britain. 4. Mentally
handicapped–Institutional care–Great Britain. 5. Mentally
handicapped–Abuse of–Great Britain. 6. Aged–Institutional
care–Great Britain. 7. Aged–Abuse of–Great Britain.
I. Stanley, Nicky, 1955–. II. Manthorpe, Jill, 1955–.
III. Penhale, Bridget, 1955–.
HV63.G7I57 1999   99–17045
362.73'2'0941–dc21   CIP

ISBN 0–415–18701–X (hbk)
ISBN 0–415–18702–8 (pbk)

Contents

Tables

Contributors

Christine Barter is a Research Officer at the NSPCC and NSPCC Research Fellow at the University of Luton.

Les Bright is Deputy General Manager of Counsel and Care.

Hilary Brown is Professor of Social Care, School of Health and Social Welfare at the Open University.

Roger Clough is Professor of Social Work at Lancaster University.

Jeanette Copperman is a freelance researcher, writer and trainer in mental health. She is a founder member of the Women and Mental Health Network.

Frank Glendenning is Honorary Senior Research Fellow, Centre for Social Gerontology at Keele University.

Frank Keating is Lecturer in Mental Health at the Tizard Centre, University of Kent.

Mary MacLeod is Director of Policy, Research and Information at ChildLine.

Julie McNamara is a survivor of the mental health services and a campaigner on mental health issues. She is a member of the Steering Group of the Women and Mental Health Network, and she is the Director of London Disability Arts Forum.

Jill Manthorpe is Senior Lecturer in Community Care at the University of Hull.

Bridget Penhale is Lecturer in Social Work at the University of Hull.

Nicky Stanley is Lecturer in Social Work at the University of Hull.

Jennie Williams is Senior Lecturer in Mental Health at the Tizard Centre, University of Kent.

Foreword

There can be no doubt about the existence of the institutional abuse of some of the most vulnerable people in society. Also, there can be no doubting the harm it has done or the way it has blighted many lives. The only doubt is the extent of it. There can be few greater responsibilities than taking on the parenting of other people's children. When the State takes on this task, the very least which should be expected is that the children will be safe from harm. It is shocking that, over the years, so many young people experience abuse whilst in public care. The danger is not confined to residential homes but can happen in foster care, adoption and in educational establishments. And it is not confined to young people. Many adults, including those with learning disabilities, those with mental health problems and vulnerable older people are potentially at risk. So the messages from this timely book should be applied widely across the caring services.

The authors have brought together contributors from research and from those with a wide range of knowledge and experience of the care system. It is particularly valuable to hear from those who have stories to tell based on their personal experiences.

It is not always acknowledged that residential work is both skilful and very demanding. The staff have to live the values which underpin good practice every minute they are on duty, when they are tired, anxious or uncertain as well as when things are going well. Residents may bring with them the hurt, disappointments and anger from their previous experiences. It is not surprising that they are often upset and disruptive, or that their behaviour can be very challenging.

Added to this, residential services for both children and adults have often been under-valued. Staff frequently receive little or no training. Supervision and support can be patchy and the most difficult situations often occur outside normal office hours, adding to the general sense of isolation. The Government deserves credit for at long last tackling the needs for residential care to be accorded a correct status and for staff to be given better training opportunities. Above all, society needs to recognise that institutional care is a vitally important part of the spectrum of services and offers the placement of positive choice for some people at a particular point in their lives. It must provide both safety and good quality care.

There is no going back to the large geographically isolated institutions of the past. Nor is it realistic to operate such small units which are not only uneconomic but also result in staff being on duty on their own. The modern unit needs to be large enough to provide a range of facilities and flexibility but not so large as to be impersonal and stigmatising. Good residential care is based upon the following:

- a clear set of values which can be translated by staff into each contact with a resident,
- a clear statement of purpose of each home,
- the building and staffing closely related to that purpose,
- an individual assessment and care plan agreed with each resident,
- regular reviews against agreed indicators of progress or deterioration,
- good record-keeping as an essential of quality care,
- regular and effective staff supervision,
- adequate training including induction training,
- ambition for the residents and the home,
- openness, honesty and constant vigilance, courage in tackling inappropriate behaviour,
- an annual audit, at least, and
- a lifetime of learning.

The latter provides the clearest justification for this important book and the contribution it makes to our understanding of the complex nature of institutional care services.

Lord Laming
October 1998

Introduction

Bridget Penhale

The abuse of individuals receiving care in institutions is not a new phenomenon. However, institutional abuse can be said to have been rediscovered in the late twentieth century in the UK and it is no longer possible to consign such abuse to the past. Reports of abuse in institutions have appeared frequently in the media in the last fifteen years but have often been superficially covered. It is nevertheless increasingly recognised that abuse is part of the experience of many residents in a number of different settings and that such abuse may be both widespread and systematic.

This volume has approached the subject matter of abuse within institutions from a different standpoint to that generally taken. The book examines institutional abuse across the life course. There are three distinct sections to the book: the first explores the situation of children living in children's homes and boarding schools; the second considers the experiences of adults with learning disabilities and adults with mental health problems; while the final section examines the position of older people who live in residential or nursing homes. This focus on abuse across the life course allows for an identification of the similarities and differences between experiences of and responses to institutional abuse for children, young adults and older adults in receipt of institutional care.

The editors considered that it was essential in a book examining institutional care to include the perspectives of the users of those services, many of whom may be considered as survivors of abuse. In each section, therefore, we have included a chapter that presents user perspectives. The value of the testimonies and accounts provided by service users is particularly evident within these chapters (by Mary MacLeod, Jeanette Copperman and Julie McNamara, Jill Manthorpe, and Les Bright) but is echoed by the other contributors to the volume. The views of users and relatives have rarely been adequately represented in inquiries into abuse. The accounts presented here emphasise the impact that such experiences have, and continue to have, on individuals. The testimonies also serve to highlight the differences between the perceptions of service users and those of professionals and policy makers involved in the field.

This book considers institutions that provide care, protection and sometimes treatment for individuals. In these places, the duty of care is of paramount concern, and when abuse occurs in such settings, it conflicts directly with the institution's stated function. As a recent report in relation to children comments:

> It may not seem realistic to expect life away from home to be safer than life at home for the generality of children. The law, however, expects it to be as safe: people caring for other people's children are required to exercise parental responsibility.
>
> (Utting 1997: 16)

By contrast, in penal settings, definitions of abuse need to be constructed in the light of rather different institutional objectives such as crime prevention, control and punishment. Care, while still relevant, becomes of lesser concern in such institutions. Penal institutions are therefore not covered here: the focus is on settings that offer care and protection.

However, those in institutional care settings may find themselves subject to high levels of control and may experience themselves as situated anywhere on the long continuum stretching from choice to coercion. It is widely assumed, in these days of post community care implementation, that the majority of adults who live in residential care are there by choice. This is of course not the case for those individuals who are committed to psychiatric or Special Hospitals under the provisions of the Mental Health Act, 1983. It is arguable, moreover, that the majority of children who are looked after within residential settings (as opposed to boarding school provision) are not there through absolute choice and that decisions have often been taken on their behalf. Both Chapters 1 and 2 make this point in relation to children's experiences of residential care.

Similarly, some older people may still experience a lack of real choice when faced with the rationing devices of local authorities in assessing their needs. Authorities may spout rhetoric concerning increased choice for individuals, yet construct such stringent eligibility criteria, particularly in relation to service provision once needs have been assessed, that the individual experiences limited or false choice.

Entry into residential or, perhaps more frequently, nursing-home care may often occur through lack of realistic and (economically) viable alternatives for individuals to remain in the environments of their choice.

Definitions and meanings

The definition of abuse remains an area for debate. There has not been any agreement between either researchers or, in the United States, legislators, as to what constitutes abuse and neglect; it is therefore difficult to extrapolate fixed truths about the incidence, prevalence and other characteristics of the phenomenon from the research findings. Nor is it certain how well such findings travel cross-culturally. Furthermore, much of the research tends to involve abuse situated within the family setting, and uses fairly small, unrepresentative samples of survivors. Many studies do not include any control group so that there are methodological difficulties in the way that the research is conducted and in the validity of the interpretation of the results.

There is also considerable controversy surrounding such issues as the definition of institutional abuse, indicators of abuse and the role of neglect within considerations of abuse. In many respects, research in this area is still in its infancy in the UK. Owing to the lack of any overall national research strategy, small-scale studies continue to be undertaken in the absence of any agreement as to the continued usefulness of such an approach. There is consequently a heavy and perhaps disproportionate emphasis on the evidence of inquiries into institutional abuse in the UK, and a number of inquiry reports will be considered in this volume.

In the absence of a standard definition of abuse, public inquiries into institutional abuse employ differing definitions, many of which have emerged from the process of one particular inquiry. Whilst the use of differing definitions need not be problematic (Penhale 1993), it is important that there is some clarity from the outset concerning what definition is being used when and for what purposes. Within public inquiries, the relationship between the members of the inquiry, the professionals involved, the individual service users and the presence of the media may interact to produce a definition of abuse for that particular inquiry. Definitions should seek to draw some distinction between individual acts by abusers within institutions, abusive regimes and examples of poor, or indeed bad practice of management and care, that is of organisational and structural problems within the institution in which abuse occurs (Bennett *et al.* 1997; Utting 1997).

It is instructive to consider the main similarities and differences between abuse that occurs within institutions and that which occurs within the domestic setting. It is, of course, critical that care in families is not idealised and romanticised; it is apparent that family life is dangerous for a significant number of individuals and bad for the health of a very large number of others (Straus *et al.* 1980). However, power relations are central to all abusive situations. What needs to be considered are the dynamics and variables that inform the abuse of power within different settings.

Structural factors, including the potential roles of gender, race, disability and age, are clearly of major importance. Considerations of gender are of particular relevance in relation to sexual and physical forms of abuse that are predominantly perpetrated by men. Race is also a pertinent structural factor within many situations of institutional abuse. Factors regarding disability are highly relevant, and some analyses emphasise vulnerability, which may itself be an oppressive or enlightening concept. Many of the models of causation that have been developed in relation to institutional abuse have tended to focus on perpetrators and their associated pathology: the so-called 'bad apple' approach (Biggs *et al.* 1995).

Consequently, the identification of and responses to abuse in institutional settings have tended to focus on flushing out individual abusers and other, arguably more critical, factors have not been accorded sufficient attention. Factors that concern wider structural oppressions and inequalities clearly need much more detailed consideration than hitherto. A number of the chapters in this volume consider in some detail the dynamics of gender, disability and the power relations that inform these dynamics.

Issues of the betrayal of trust and of the reification of secrecy are also found in both abuse within families and in that within institutions. However, the nature of betrayal in institutional abuse differs as the concept of trust differs. Trust involves a complex web of relationships and is derived from the care contract. This care contract is crucial in distinguishing abuse in institutions from abuse in families.

The role and nature of the care contract between the institution and the service user has both explicit and implicit elements. It may, of course, be less explicit for some groups than for others: for example, children and mental health service users may not be signatories to a contract. Recent statements by the Department of Health in relation to 'corporate parenting' (Secretary of State for Health 1998) may be seen as attempts to make the contract more explicit in relation to children. However, within the field of learning disabilities and in the care of older people, contractual arrangements are much more likely to be used. This is especially evident in relation to those individuals who are in receipt of assistance via public funding for their care, when the contract is likely to include the local authority as a party. It may be the case that the formal contract that is established in such instances is essentially between the local authority and the provider (the institution) rather than with the individual who receives the care. In these instances the individual service user is not a signatory to the contract in any formal sense.

We can discern the existence of rather more implicit and informal contracts between the individual service user and the provider, and between the local authority (or health purchaser) and the individual. It is possible to conceptualise this contract as being triangular in form: between the service user, the provider (institution) and the State (as purchaser and regulator of care). Such contracts, whether implicit or explicit, charge the institution with a duty of care with regard to individuals who are vulnerable. The existence of abuse within such settings can be viewed as a failure to ensure that the duty of care is upheld and can be conceptualised as a violation of the implicit terms of the contract.

A further distinction between familial abuse and abuse within institutional settings is found in the relationship between individual service users. While residents of institutions live together, often in conditions of some intimacy that approximate to family life, they will not necessarily be in close or intimate relationships with one another. However, as the chapters by Nicky Stanley, Hilary Brown and Jennie Williams and Frank Keating confirm, there is increasing recognition of the abuse that occurs between residents in institutions. In addition, within institutional settings there may also be risks of abuse being directed by residents at members of staff or at relatives (Department of Health and Social Services Inspectorate 1996).

When considering definitions, meanings and understandings, it is also relevant to look briefly at what we understand by the term 'institution'. As with abuse, there is no standard definition of an institution. Dictionary definitions provide a number of different meanings for the word. Institution may mean a society or organisation. The word concerns structure, function and process, not merely the presence of a physical entity or building (Jack 1998). In a recent exploration of residential provision, Jack suggests that the term institution has become synonymous with a particular form of service provision and processes of institutionalisation. He argues that a somewhat simplistic, dualistic concept can be identified within both public and professional arenas, and suggests that this concept equates community with good care and institutions with all that is bad. Whilst Jack is surely correct to challenge such over-simplifications, his alternative model that contrasts neglect in the community with high quality residential care appears equally misleading. It is notable that his analysis fails to include any detailed consideration of institutional abuse.

For the purposes of this volume, institution refers to care provided within a home that is not owned by the individual, and where the locus of control lies beyond the individual living in that environment. Also central to the definition is that the individual lives with others and there is often likely to be little or no choice as to who those individuals are. Control over the structure, function and organisation of the home is not within the power of the individual but is exercised by members of staff who are not ordinarily resident in that environment. Indeed, the extent of control, or lack of control, by individuals in relation to their living environment appears to be a key defining element of an institution, although the degree of control available to them is likely to vary between different settings.

Much of the care within institutional settings is valuable, of good quality and provided well. An unnecessary polarisation between community living as first choice and institutional care as last resort seems evident in many recent statements about institutional care. This has not been assisted by much of the rhetoric surrounding the implementation of the community care reforms, which tended to imply that community provision was the only appropriate form of care that is relevant for individuals.

However, in eschewing the over-simplified conflict model of community care versus institutions, we must not ignore the testaments of service users in general, and of survivors of institutional abuse in particular. Such testaments tend to affirm a view that care in community settings is more desirable for individuals than continuing long-term care in institutions, particularly if those settings are ones in which abuse occurs and in some instances is perpetuated.

A number of approaches have been taken in relation to establishing definitions of institutional abuse. Such abuse can be conceived of as existing at three different levels. The following schema can be used to structure the concept of institutional abuse:

- Level 1: abuse between individuals within the residential setting;
- Level 2: abuse arising due to the regime of the institution;
- Level 3: abuse arising at a system level (broader social structure).

This type of approach is also suggested within Gil's (1982) work, which identified three different forms of institutional abuse in relation to children. The first form was the overt or direct abuse of a child by a care worker. The abuse could be physical, sexual or emotional, or indeed there could be multiple forms of abuse in co-existence. The second form of institutional abuse identified by Gil was termed 'Programme Abuse' and referred to the existence of an abusive regime or treatment programme within an institution. The 'Pindown' regime that existed within Staffordshire Social Services in the 1980s and that is more fully discussed in Chapter 1 is an example of this type.

The third form of abuse is that of 'System Abuse'. This corresponds to the third level, that of the broader social system. In Gil's terms it refers to abuse that is perpetrated and perpetuated by the system and in which the safety of individuals within institutional care cannot be guaranteed (1982). By altering the first part of Gil's definition from child to individual, it is possible to consider the definition of institutional abuse in a rather more holistic way than simply considering either the different types of abuse or the range of settings in which abuse occurs.

The changing context of institutional care

In exploring institutional abuse, it is necessary to acknowledge the changing nature of institutions and the care provided by them. These recent changes form part of structural changes in welfare provision in the UK.

The 1960s and 1970s witnessed the flourishing of the movement towards community care and the provision of care to individuals in their own homes. This was coupled with the development of views concerning the detrimental effects of institutional life and 'batch living' on individuals. The union of the two strands resulted in a strong and healthy infant: care in the community with associated changes in social policy acting as midwives in attendance. These policy changes took place together with legislative change in the form of the NHS and Community Care Act, 1990 that was finally fully implemented in 1993. This framework has seen the further development of the perception of institutions as places of last resort, and the range and scope of institutional care has been altered as a consequence.

In recent decades, there has been an overall decrease in the number of institutions in the public sector and a rise in the number of institutions for adults that are run by the private or not for profit (including the voluntary) sector (Peace *et al.* 1997). We have witnessed the closure of a large number of children's homes and of traditional psychiatric hospitals (Gooch 1996; Goodwin 1997). Institutions are generally smaller in size and more diverse in terms of their provision: for example, the amount of respite care provision has increased (Moriarty and Levin 1998; Stalker 1996). They are less likely to be socially or geographically isolated and many residential homes are now more integrated into the communities in which they are located. The growth of residential homes offering care to a very small number of residents who may in some instances actually be considered as part of a family (Holland and Peace 1998) further contributes to an increasingly diverse sector. Such homes can still be considered institutions by virtue of their organisational setting in which care is provided and finance is exchanged.

Goffman's (1961) seminal work on institutions continues to form a backcloth to our understanding of institutions but needs to be re-examined in the context of this changing social environment. Goffman's work involved the construction of a model of the 'total institution' and he explored the processes of de-personalisation that individuals experienced in such institutions. Routine served as an example of the process that shaped this experience. While he presented an overview of the institution, it is often forgotten that he argued for a fivefold classification. This included:

- institutions designed to care for the 'incapable and harmless' (e.g. homes for the 'blind, aged or orphaned');
- institutions established to care for the 'incapable', who present an unintended threat to the community (e.g. sanatoria; mental hospitals);
- institutions organised to protect the community from 'intentional dangers' (e.g. prisons);
- institutions established for some 'work-like task' (e.g. army barracks; boarding schools);
- institutions set up as retreats from the world (e.g. monasteries).

Such classifications may be increasingly blurred but it is with the first two types that this book is principally concerned, although there is some consideration of boarding schools (type four above) in relation to the institutional abuse of young people. For Goffman, it was possible to identify common characteristics of institutions that might be present, albeit to varying degrees. Essentially, the key features of total institutions were:

First, all aspects of life are conducted in the same place, and under the same single authority. Second, each phase of the members' daily activity is carried on in the immediate company of a large batch of others, all of whom are treated alike and required to do the same thing together. Third, all phases of the day's activities are tightly scheduled with one activity leading at a pre-arranged time into the next, the whole sequence of activities being imposed from above by a system of explicit formal rulings and a body of officials.

(Goffman 1961: 17)

Thus, in Goffman's view, it was the fundamental nature of institutions and institutional care that led to a degradation of care. He argued that the removal of normal, everyday patterns of activity and identities for individuals constituted the essence of institutional life. Within this specific context the individual is de-personalised. Wardhaugh and Wilding's exploration of the corruption of care develops this concept of de-personalisation to argue that if individuals are viewed as less than human and 'not like us', then abuse of those individuals becomes more explicable, if not justifiable (1993).

In recent years there has been some criticism of Goffman's work, arguing that his account failed to examine the relationship between the institution and the broader social context (Perring 1992). As noted, a number of the chapters in this book argue that social identity, as defined by gender, disability, race and age, informs the dynamics of institutional abuse. Recent theory emphasises the centrality of the body in the construction of identity, and we would therefore suggest that while those receiving institutional care may be disempowered, structural factors such as gender, disability and race continue to shape abusive interactions within institutions. While Goffman's concept of de-personalisation now seems limited, his work continues to provide a vivid and persuasive account of the role of power inequalities in defining institutional life.

Few current institutions fit within Goffman's original definition of a total institution. For example, generally not all aspects of life are carried out in one place (young people attend school; occupation or training may be provided for adults); not all activities are carried out by all individuals at the same time, nor are all aspects of the regime rigidly programmed at all times. The move towards smaller community-based institutions may suggest a fundamental change in the nature of institutional care, but this may only be a superficial change. Smaller institutions often lack the elaborate hierarchies that made it so difficult to achieve change in the larger institutions. It may also mean that it is easier to intervene to achieve change and that the boundaries between the home and the community are more permeable. However, in some instances the institution may be owned by the person responsible for the daily management of the unit, which can present particular areas of difficulty. It is arguable, too, that in smaller units the balance of power and the opportunities for abuse of that power remain potentially problematic. Within smaller institutions, however, the population of residents and staff may change more frequently than in larger, more traditionally run, units. The chapters by Hilary Brown and Jill Manthorpe identify such issues in relation to an inquiry into the care of people with learning disabilities in one particular home.

It is appropriate to add that many institutions now do not stand alone, but increasingly work in partnership with other forms of care provision. The potential partnerships with short-term provision such as respite care and fostering, or schemes where residential and nursing homes provide day and domiciliary care services to older people within the locality may be indicative of future options. Residential homes have also been developing a much more person-centred and 'homely' style of provision (Holland and Peace 1998). There have been moves to make residential homes more open, with links to communities, families and the neighbourhood.

Therein lies a challenge: how to provide a home that is more 'homely' yet also more open to public scrutiny and regulatory mechanisms in a way in which domestic homes are not. The existence of smaller homes that are more integrated into the local community does not necessarily mean that the home will be more open or free from abuse or abusive practices. Families have traditionally not been particularly open to outside scrutiny, given the historical and societal perspectives that linger concerning the right to privacy and freedom from public interference in what are considered 'private matters' for the family to deal with.

As many of the contributors to this book argue, the response to institutional abuse is not just about improving care standards. Awareness of the possibility of abuse occurring within institutions and the risk factors involved can affect decisions about the provision of care, and, for individuals, decisions about choice of care. Within the field of child care, the publicised failure of care provided in some residential homes and schools, together with scandals relating to abuse within such settings has led to an increasing loss of public confidence in the ability of such homes to provide safety and protection for their residents. This has been coupled with a growing concern that there may not exist an absolute place of safety for young people.

Developments that are currently taking place or are anticipated – such as an independent inspectorate for residential care and nursing homes; the introduction of the General Social Care Council and Government initiatives concerning caring for children and young people in residential care homes (Secretary of State for Health 1998); and the protection of vulnerable adults in care homes – may go some way toward restoring confidence. It will take some time, however, for the public to feel sufficiently assured that residential care is anything other than a last resort for individuals who need care, and this may in itself be a key factor in the development and perpetuation of abuse within institutions.

The structure of the book

The eleven chapters in this book deal with a range of different residential institutions, but all share a common concern: to examine the various forms that abuse in institutional settings may take for particular groups of individuals. As described above, the book has taken a life course approach so that all the chapters fall into one of the three main stages of the life course: childhood, adulthood or later life.

Chapter 1, by Nicky Stanley, provides an overview of the abuse of children in residential settings. The chapter considers past and recent inquiries into abuse and the ensuing Government response in the UK as well as relevant research. The nature of abuse is explored in relation to issues of control and restraint, gender and sexuality, bullying and institutional abuse. Some of the key developments that constitute a response to abuse are discussed.

The perspectives of children concerning abuse in institutional settings are examined in Chapter 2 through Mary MacLeod's analysis of calls made to ChildLine's telephone helpline. Experiences of abuse in both residential care and educational settings (boarding schools) are discussed and some first-person accounts are included. The descriptions by the young people cover a wide range of different forms of abuse occurring within such settings. Consideration is also given to the types of support available to assist young people who experience such abuse.

Chapter 3, by Christine Barter, describes an NSPCC research study of investigations into child abuse in institutional settings and sets this study against a background of research findings from the United States. The study considers the problems associated with such investigations and suggests some possible solutions. This chapter also examines the support needs of both young people and members of staff during the course of investigations, and a useful protocol for investigations is outlined.

The next chapter, by Hilary Brown, opens the sections covering the institutional care of adults. It explores the extent of abuse amongst adults with learning disabilities within institutional care and relates this to research findings in the UK and other countries. The chapter provides an overview of vulnerability factors in relation to adults with learning disabilities and also considers philosophies of care and the appropriate legal context. The results of one particular inquiry into institutional abuse are presented as a case study in this complex and sensitive area.

Chapter 5, by Jill Manthorpe, focuses on the perspectives and involvement of service users in this area. Consideration is also given to the views of caregivers, and the role of campaigning and advocacy services in general is examined in some depth. Dr Ann Craft had agreed to write this chapter but her untimely death meant that a substitute was needed and we are fortunate that Jill was able to assist with this. The work of Dr Craft and the organisation that she helped to set up, NAPSAC, now renamed the Ann Craft Trust, have been central to developing understanding and good practice in this area and her early death has both diminished the field and provoked much sadness.

The following two chapters, 6 and 7, consider the abuse of adults in mental health settings. This is an area that receives little coverage in the media and where public awareness is generally low. Special Hospitals are today the institutions that most closely resemble Goffman's total institution. In Chapter 6, Jennie Williams and Frank Keating provide an overview, considering the factors involved in the abuse of individuals within mental health settings. In particular, the extent to which such abuse mirrors social inequalities is examined. This chapter includes findings from recent studies of adults with mental health problems and identifies the difficulties experienced by mental health service users in voicing experiences of abuse.

Chapter 7, by Jeanette Copperman and Julie McNamara, presents the voices of survivors of abuse in mental health settings, with particular focus on the sexual abuse that many women patients experience. Abuse in relation to treatment regimes and consent to treatment is also addressed within this somewhat bleak, yet moving collection of accounts.

The final sequence of three chapters is concerned with the abuse of older people within residential and nursing care settings. Frank Glendenning provides an overview account of this area in Chapter 8. Current knowledge and findings from relevant research in both the United States and the UK are brought together here. Although the focus of the chapter is on residential and nursing homes, the range of settings in which institutional abuse occurs is covered and recommendations for future work and practice are explored.

Chapter 9, by Les Bright, is concerned with the experiences of older people within institutional care and also provides accounts from caregivers. The chapter draws on work recently undertaken by the voluntary organisation, Counsel and Care, in response to a range of different types of abuse and abusive situations that have been identified within institutional settings for older people. Attention is given to the factors that contribute to abusive regimes and to a lack of respect for individuals who live in such care settings.

The final chapter in this sequence, by Roger Clough, focuses on the role of management and of regulatory and inspection mechanisms in relation to residential and nursing-home settings. This draws on Professor Clough's extensive experience as Chief Inspector of a Local Authority Social Services Department Registration and Inspection Unit. The part played by such mechanisms in identifying and defining situations of abuse and neglect is examined and proposals outlining good practice in this area are included.

Chapter 11, by Jill Manthorpe and Nicky Stanley, acts as a conclusion and draws together the major themes of the book. Similarities and differences in abuse across the life course are examined, as are issues in connection with professional whistle-blowing, abuse prevention and training. This final chapter returns to the themes of users' voices and suggests that the concept of users' rights may offer a framework for combating abuse and the attitudes that feed it.

The original ideas for the book arose from discussions between the editors in 1997 concerning different forms of institutional abuse and its impact on groups of service users. We identified a need to compare and contrast these experiences, drawing on the vivid accounts provided by users. Only by increasing our knowledge and understanding in this way will we be able to begin to develop really effective strategies for the prevention of abuse across the life course. The commitment and enthusiasm of the contributors to this project has reinforced our conviction concerning the value of this approach.

The wider phenomenon of interpersonal violence is a social problem that is increasingly recognised. Within the study of interpersonal violence, the issue of institutional abuse, in all the forms that it takes, needs to be subject to a careful analysis that probes behind the sensationalist headlines and defensive responses that characterise discussions of abuse in the public arena. It is with this goal in mind that this book has been put together. We trust that the resulting volume goes some way towards achieving that goal.

References

Bennett, G., Kingston, P. and Penhale, B. (1997) *The Dimensions of Elder Abuse*, Basingstoke: Macmillan.

Biggs, S., Phillipson, C. and Kingston, P. (1995) *Elder Abuse in Perspective*, Basingstoke: Macmillan.

Department of Health and Social Services Inspectorate (1996) *Responding to Residents*, London: HMSO.

Gil, E. (1982) 'Institutional abuse of children in out-of-home care', in R. Hanson (ed.) *Institutional Abuse of Children and Youth*, New York: Haworth Press.

Goffman, E. (1961) *Asylums: Essays on the Social Situation of Mental Patients and Other Inmates*, New York: Anchor/Doubleday.

Gooch, D. (1996) 'Home and away: the residential care, education and control of children in historical and political context', *Child and Family Social Work* 1: 19–32.

Goodwin, S. (1997) *Comparative Mental Health Policy*, London: Sage.

Holland, C. and Peace, S. (1998) *Homely Residential Care: Report of a Pilot Study of Small Homes for Older People Carried Out in Bedfordshire, Buckinghamshire and Hertfordshire During 1997*, Milton Keynes: Open University Press.

Jack, R. (ed.) (1998) *Residential Versus Community Care*, Basingstoke: Macmillan.

Moriarty, J. and Levin, E. (1998) 'Respite care in homes and hospitals', in R. Jack (ed.) *Residential Versus Community Care*, Basingstoke: Macmillan.

Peace, S., Kellaher, L. and Willcocks, D. (1997) *Re-evaluating Residential Care*, Buckingham: Open University Press.

Penhale, B. (1993) 'The abuse of elderly people: considerations for practice', *British Journal of Social Work* 23(2): 95–112.

Perring, C. (1992) 'The experience and perspectives of patients and care staff of the transition from hospital to community based care', in S. Ramon (ed.) *Psychiatric Hospital Closure: Myths and Realities*, London: Chapman Hall.

Secretary of State for Health (1998) *The Government's Response to the Children's Safeguards Review*, Cmd 4105, London: HMSO.

Stalker, K. (ed.) (1996) *Developments in Short-Term Care*, London: Jessica Kingsley.

Straus, M., Gelles, R. and Steinmetz, S. (1980) *Behind Closed Doors: Violence in the American Family*, New York: Anchor/Doubleday.

Utting, W. (1997) *People Like Us: The Report of the Review of the Safeguards for Children Living Away from Home*, London: The Stationery Office.

Wardhaugh, J. and Wilding, P. (1993) 'Towards an explanation of the corruption of care', *Journal of Social Policy* 37: 4–31.

1 The institutional abuse of children

An overview of policy and practice

Nicky Stanley

The abuse of children in residential settings has sprung to the fore of public consciousness in the 1990s through a series of inquiries and court cases that have been reported in detail by the media. The press and television coverage has served to bring the often vivid testimonies of those who experienced abuse in places where they might have expected to feel safe to the attention of a large audience, and has exposed both local authorities and voluntary organisations to the charge of failing to protect those most in need of care. The identification of residential care as a locus for the abuse of children has led to a crisis of confidence that is not confined to residential services for children, but has spread to embrace child protection services as a whole. The Government has responded to this crisis with a series of policy initiatives backed up by exhortations to social services departments and local politicians to meet identified targets (Secretary of State for Health 1998; Department of Health 1998a). At the level of practice, concerns about abuse in out-of-home-care settings can have the effect of making the use of care orders seem as risky a strategy as leaving children in abusive home situations.

Not only has public confidence in the capacity of residential care to protect children been undermined, but the whole concept of institutional care for children appears alien to the current orthodoxy of child care theory. The Children Act, 1989 explicitly identifies 'normal family life' (Department of Health 1989: 8) in the birth family as the ideal system of care, and places duties on local authorities to promote the care of children by their families. Gooch points out that the decline in the popularity of residential care for children has a long history and argues that residence has long been a 'pragmatic' rather than an ideological response to poverty (Gooch 1996: 25).

In the absence of a supportive ideology, residential care for children, long characterised as a poor relation, has become an increasingly marginalised service and the influential Government review, *People Like Us* (Utting 1997), notes the shrinkage of places in residential homes from 40,000 children in 1975 to 8,000 in 1995. This sharp drop is explained in part by an overall reduction in the numbers of children looked after by English local authorities but also by the development of foster care services, which have suffered only a slight decrease in numbers by comparison (Berridge 1997). However, it is also important to recognise the phenomenon of the increasingly fast turnover of places in residential homes. Berridge and Brodie's (1998) two-part study of children's homes allows for a comparison of the characteristics of two sample populations with a ten-year gap between them. They found a reduction in the average length of stay in the current home from nearly two years in 1985 to ten months in 1995. While the average length of stay in care had dropped significantly between the two samples, the children in the 1995 sample were still experiencing multiple placements, with adolescents being particularly likely to have had more than one residential placement (Berridge and Brodie 1998). Berridge and Brodie also note that a sixth of the total population of children's homes are placed there on respite care. While the number of places in residential homes have clearly shrunk dramatically, large numbers of children are passing through them.

Boarding schools now represent the largest form of institutional provision for children with 110,000 places in England and Wales in 1996 (Utting 1997). Eighty thousand of these are in independent boarding schools where children have been placed by their parents', if not their own, choice. The remaining places are mainly in boarding schools for children with special needs, the majority of whom are placed there by local authorities. While the number of children boarding in independent schools has declined significantly over the last twenty years, the reduction is less steep in the number of places in special boarding schools. Gooch (1996) argues that the underlying trend behind these changes is a shift to children entering boarding school at a later stage so that boarding in special schools is now virtually confined to children of secondary-school age. He notes also the success of the independent day schools in mounting a challenge to the hegemony of the independent boarding school. However, Utting (1997) points out that, in respect of special boarding schools, the numbers in local authority and voluntary establishments (which together provide 84 per cent of the sector) have changed little in recent years and are unlikely to do so.

This chapter will focus primarily on institutional care in children's homes, since it is this sector that has given rise to most of the accounts of abuse. The number of children accommodated in secure units is small: 246 at March 1996 (Utting 1997). However, such units, which are run by local authorities for children likely to cause serious injury to themselves or others, are of particular importance when the issue of bullying is under discussion. Boarding schools have also been the subject of some major inquiries and the children in special boarding schools might be considered particularly vulnerable to abuse. Utting (1997) comments on the lack of evidence concerning children in adolescent and mental health units. While Westcott (1991a) has usefully collated some of the American research into the institutional abuse of children, much of the evidence in the United Kingdom is derived from inquiry reports although ChildLine's telephone line service has produced an impressive series of accounts from children themselves (see Chapter 2 in this volume). This chapter will discuss some of the major inquiries and reviews before looking in more detail at the current nature of institutional care for children. A number of issues arising from accounts of institutional abuse will be considered; these will cover, first, aspects of abuse and, second, responses to institutional abuse.

Inquiry reports and reviews

Over the last ten years a pattern has emerged whereby the public outrage evoked by media reporting of cases of institutional abuse is assuaged, first, by an inquiry into the institution concerned and, second, by a Government review providing a broader context for the inquiry and recommending new policy initiatives. The Pindown Inquiry attracted a high level of public attention and the inquiry team were appointed in the immediate wake of a Granada Television programme in 1990 that featured the system used to control children in a number of residential homes in Staffordshire in the 1980s. The inquiry report (Levy and Kahan 1991) provides detailed accounts of 'Pindown' that entailed the isolation of children, the removal of their clothes and personal possessions, and the loss of direct access to education, leisure and hygiene facilities. The architect of the system, which appears to have been based on a very crude understanding of behavioural programmes, was Tony Latham, a trained social worker who rose to the position of Area Manager in the social services hierarchy. His methods were readily adopted by those who worked in institutions that he managed and were open to scrutiny by managers who found nothing to criticise.

The inquiry report was unequivocal in judging the 'isolation, humiliation and confrontation' of children that Pindown entailed to be 'intrinsically unethical, unprofessional and unacceptable' (Levy and Kahan 1991: 127). Middle management was heavily criticised in the report and, as well as a number of procedural recommendations, issues concerning staffing policies, supervision and training for basic-grade workers were given prominence.

The inquiry report resulted in the Government commissioning Sir William Utting's first review of residential childcare. This review, *Children in the Public Care* (Utting 1991), was confined to England, but companion reviews were undertaken in Wales (Social Services Inspectorate, Wales and Social Information Systems 1991) and Scotland (Skinner 1992). These reviews acknowledge residential care's role as a residual service: Utting's definition of the task of residential homes for children makes it clear that the main role of the service is to back up foster care. Residential care's purpose is to provide a home for children who

• have decided that they do not wish to be fostered;
• have had bad experiences of foster care;
• have been so abused within the family that another family placement is inappropriate;
• are from the same family and cannot otherwise be kept together.

(Utting, 1991: 8)

The review of children's homes in Wales was even more explicit in describing residential care for children as 'a marginal unspecific activity taking those whose needs the rest of the system fails to meet' (Social Services Inspectorate, Wales and Social Information Systems 1991: 11). This report proposed that a clear distinction should be made between homes for children displaying challenging behaviour and homes for those whose need for residential care was based on circumstance rather than behaviour. While confirming that residential care for children was in decline, Utting asserted that residential care was, nevertheless, an 'indispensable service' (Utting 1991: 62) and a similarly revivalist tone is discernible in the Scottish review's argument that residential childcare should be seen as 'a positive means of meeting the needs of particular children, not simply as a last resort' (Skinner 1992). Kahan, in *Growing Up in Groups* (1994), a publication that sprang out of an interprofessional working group that aimed to define good practice, identifies a call to reintegrate residential child care into mainstream services as a common message of all three reviews.

In 1991 Frank Beck received five life sentences for sexual and physical assaults against children in homes in Leicestershire between 1973 and 1986. These included offences of buggery and rape. The inquiry chaired by Andrew Kirkwood QC reported in 1993 and found that many complaints had been made over a number of years concerning physical and sexual assaults, and the 'regression therapy' practised by Beck and his staff. This 'therapy' involved the humiliation and aggressive confrontation of children in order to provoke angry tantrums that were responded to with physical restraint. The report attributes the failure of social services managers to respond to these complaints to 'A general predisposition not to believe children', an 'out of sight, out of mind' attitude and a fear of challenging Beck on the grounds of his claims to expertise and to the irreplaceability of his service (Kirkwood 1993: 312).

Both Pindown and the regime promoted by Beck provide illustrations of the way in which theoretical labels and concepts were used to confer credibility and intellectual respectability on abusive practices. It seems as though a few vague references to theoretical models, derived in the one case from learning theory, in the other from the psychoanalytic tradition, were sufficient to reassure managers and other professionals (which in Beck's case included psychiatrists) that the radical model of care employed constituted sound and effective practice. Social work's relationship to theory has always been problematic and the translation of psychological theory into social work practice has at times entailed crude appropriation rather than informed application of complex theoretical models. However, as Payne (1997) notes, the theoretical base of residential social work is particularly undeveloped by comparison with other forms of social work and much of the residential care literature is pragmatic rather than theoretical in its approach. This theoretical vacuum allows pseudo-theories to go unchallenged. The Kirkwood report also stresses the lack of childcare expertise and knowledge among Beck's managers.

The committee of inquiry, established by the Secretary of State for Health in response to the conviction of Beck, reported before the inquiry report was published. Chaired by Norman Warner, the committee's remit centred on staff selection and recruitment but also embraced management and other issues. The report was also able to draw on the findings of the inquiry into Ty Mawr Community Home in Gwent (Williams and Macreadie 1992) that were published shortly before the committee reported. At Ty Mawr, the adolescent male residents appeared to be out of control and there were a worrying number of suicide attempts and incidents of self-harm. This report had drawn attention to the largely unqualified nature of the staff and identified the inappropriate involvement of elected members in the appointment of staff. The Warner report, *Choosing With Care*, identified 'low self-esteem' as a problem both for the residential sector and for the staff working there, and argued that 'Children's homes now need their place in the managerial sun' (Warner 1992: 8). The report outlined a new, comprehensive strategy for the training of staff in residential care which would embrace all levels of staff, not just officers-in-charge. The emphasis was to be on workplace-based training that would be identified and monitored through a Personal Development Contract. Warner also questioned the relevance of the traditional Diploma in Social Work curriculum for residential social work and proposed the introduction of a new diploma. The report made detailed proposals on recruitment, selection and appointment procedures for staff in residential settings.

In response to the Utting and Warner Reports, the Department of Health launched a number of initiatives that included the long-awaited review of pay in residential care (Local Government Management Board 1992) and the establishment of the Department of Health Support Force for Children's Residential Care. Measures were introduced to increase the number of professionally qualified staff in children's homes and progress was made towards defining quality standards for residential child care (Central Council for Training in Social Work [CCETSW] and Department of Health Expert Group 1992). The Government also commissioned a series of research studies into the management and practice of residential childcare, a number of which are reported on below. However, public attention since 1993 has shifted from the issue of the abusive regime to the question of the sexual abuse of children in residential settings by individuals labelled as career paedophiles.

Frank Beck remains the most notorious of these cases but the Kirkwood report had been preceded by the publication of the inquiry into the sexual abuse of children by Ralph Morris, head of Castle Hill School, a non-maintained special school in Shropshire (Brannen *et al.* 1992). This inquiry report was published, at the suggestion of the Departments of Health and Education, as a guide to good practice in such investigations. As with Beck, a number of complaints made by children from the school against Morris met with no response and the report made various recommendations concerning complaints procedures. The independent educational status of Castle Hill raised issues concerning registration and inspection procedures as well as the question of the use of the institution for placements by several different local authorities.

Since 1993, there have been a number of cases of abuse of children in institutional settings that have come to the public attention through media coverage of the investigations and trials of individuals, rather than through publications of inquiry reports. These cases have been based on allegations of abuse from adults against those who cared for them in the past. The majority of these cases have involved sexual assaults on boys and a string of convictions have resulted from a proactive police approach which has involved police forces in different parts of the United Kingdom seeking out and interviewing potential victims subsequent to an initial allegation. The investigations have identified a string of men who have been found guilty of sexually assaulting children they cared for in a number of institutions during their careers. While some of these individuals worked in the same institutions, there has as yet been no convincing evidence of 'organised abuse'. The scale of the abuse identified, that occurred in children's homes and schools in Merseyside, Cheshire, North Wales, South Wales, Doncaster and Sunderland, has been such as to prompt the comment in a broadsheet newspaper that:

> It is now clear that during the last 30 years, children's homes in Britain suffered an epidemic of rape and violent assault.
>
> (Davies 1998: 6)

The cumulative effect of this recent series of cases has been to shift the focus away from abusive regimes to a focus on the detection and control of individual paedophiles.

At the time of writing, the publication of the report of the North Wales Tribunal is imminent. The Tribunal, which sat from 1997 to 1998 under the chairmanship of Sir Ronald Waterhouse QC, was set up by Parliament in response to dissatisfactions with internal local authority inquiries and investigations. Seven men had already been convicted of offences against children in residential homes and schools in Clwyd and Gwynedd; these cases and allegations connected with them involved 650 complainants identified by the police. As a counterbalance to some of the criticisms made of police methods that relied on seeking out incriminating evidence from adults who stood to benefit from compensation claims and who themselves might have criminal convictions (Webster 1998), the Tribunal has traced and interviewed a random sample of former residents, some of whom have voluntarily added to the accounts of abuse experienced in the homes under consideration.

The Department of Health, however, had already responded to the increasing number of cases of abuse of children in out-of-home-care by commissioning a second review from Sir William Utting. The publication of *People Like Us: The Report of the Review of the Safeguards for Children Living Away from Home* in 1997 can be seen as an attempt to reassure the public at a point when the image of institutional care for children had sunk to an all-time low. Many of the messages of the review reiterate the themes of earlier reports; for instance, Warner's recommendation that the Government establish a Development Action Group for residential care for children is revived by Utting. This proposal has finally been translated into Government policy with the announcement of a Ministerial Task Force (Secretary of State for Health 1998) that will monitor the programme of action conceived in response to *People Like Us*. Utting's 1997 review includes a focus on career abusers and a concern about the low rate of convictions in cases of child sex abuse, and the review recommends the full implementation of the Advisory Group on Video-recorded Evidence (1989) on video evidence as well as a general review of the current arrangements for the prosecution of alleged sex offenders against children. Utting also argues strongly that the current level of provision in residential child-care has shrunk to the point where a child's safety cannot be assured as there is no choice of placements available, and the Social Services Inspectorate (SSI) report, *Someone Else's Children* (1998) reiterates the theme of limited placement choice. However, it may be misleading to argue that more places will result in a choice of placements being available. The high cost of places in residential care tends to have the effect of ensuring full occupancy in institutions. Sinclair and Gibbs (1998) find no reason for increasing the size of residential care provision for children and maintain that, as the main argument for residential care is that there is no alternative for those children who require it, local authorities who are managing with the current level of provision would see little reason to expand the service.

The nature of current provision

Not only has the size of the residential care sector for children changed but, in parallel with developments in adult care, private ownership of children's homes has increased while local authorities and voluntary organisations have significantly reduced the numbers of children's homes they own and manage (Brown *et al.* 1998). Berridge and Brodie (1998) note the difficulties experienced by social services managers in London seeking to monitor the quality of placements in private homes: the London borough included in their study had 210 children placed in seventy private homes outside London. In the field of special boarding schools, the majority of schools are still maintained by local authorities (Utting 1997).

It is widely accepted that the population of children's homes is now predominantly adolescent and predominantly troubled or troublesome. Utting describes these young people as 'experiencing a crisis of disordered or challenging behaviour' (1991: 9). Responding to and controlling this behaviour has become a round-the-clock job in the cases of the disproportionate numbers of children in residential care who are excluded from school (Department of Health and Office for Standards in Education 1995). In special boarding schools the population is also predominantly adolescent and boys are over-represented (Grimshaw with Berridge 1994). Questions of discipline and restraint in institutions for children have been explicitly addressed in the 1990s and these will be discussed in more detail below. However, Brown *et al.* (1998) point out that at least 15 per cent of the children in residential care are under 10 years old. Sinclair and Gibbs (1998) found that, in their sample of 176 children living in children's homes, violence was commoner amongst children under twelve and they suggest that since residential care is now perceived as a resource for adolescents, younger children who are placed there are likely to be extremely disruptive. In this study, younger children also appeared more vulnerable to bullying (Sinclair and Gibbs 1998).

There have been difficulties in estimating the numbers of disabled children in institutions (Morris 1995). However, Loughran *et al.* (1992), in their secondary analysis of the OPCS data, produced the finding that 37 per cent of children in residential homes were disabled. The growing use of residential care as a respite service has had the effect of introducing more children with disabilities into the residential care system. The increased vulnerability of this group to abuse in all settings has been well documented (Westcott 1991b; Westcott and Cross 1996), and a study of eighty-four cases known to the NSPCC of children abused in institutional settings identified 37 per cent of the children as disabled (Westcott and Clément 1992). However, since this research does not identify what proportion of the population of the institutions concerned were classified as disabled, it is difficult to assess the significance of this finding. Children with disabilities may be easily intimidated by other children – 51 per cent of perpetrators in the NSPCC study were other children – as well as by adult carers. Disabled children are put at increased risk of abuse by the involvement of multiple carers who may undertake intimate care tasks (Westcott and

Cross 1996). They may also be perceived as isolated and less likely to disclose abuse.

The rest of this chapter will look, first, at specific aspects of abuse in institutions and, second, at the range of responses to the evidence of abuse that has emerged from the inquiries and from recent research.

Aspects of abuse

Control and restraint

Control is a key feature of life in institutions: residents have to live by the timetable and rules (written and unwritten) of the institution and will incur penalties if they fail to do so. The majority of children in residential care have not consented to entering the institution; coercion therefore becomes a fundamental element in the implicit contract between child and residential establishment. This element of coercion is apparent in the responses to the survey of 2,000 looked-after children commissioned by the Who Cares? Trust (Shaw 1998). The two worst things about being in care most frequently cited by respondents were separation from family and friends, and regulations and formalities. This study also included children in foster care who were twice as likely to find nothing wrong with being looked after as were those children living in institutions.

Pindown was clearly an attempt to exert control over a group of children who were seen as prone to absconding: one of the house rules of the unit where it was employed was 'DO AS IS TOLD' (Levy and Kahan 1991: 198). Fuelled by crude ideas about therapeutic techniques, unregulated and in the hands of its exponents, this approach went disastrously 'over the top'. However, the boundary between discipline or restraint and abuse remains difficult to define and easy to cross. Berridge and Brodie (1998) found that 'control' was the issue that staff in residential children's homes found most worrying.

The Children Act 1989 Guidance and Regulations: Volume 4, Residential Care (Department of Health 1991) provides the basic guidance on issues of control and discipline, and makes it clear that corporal punishment and the use of accommodation to restrict a child's liberty physically is unacceptable (Section 1.19). Demands for more specific guidance concerning what approaches staff could use to control children's behaviour led to the Department of Health issuing in 1993, *Guidance on Permissible Forms of Control in Children's Residential Care*, which defined the circumstances under which children could be prevented from leaving the institution as those in which there were grounds for believing that the children could put themselves or others at risk and/or seriously damage property. This was followed up in 1997 by a letter from the Chief Inspector pointing out that residential care staff had the 'responsibility *and the authority* to interpret "harm" widely and to anticipate when it is clearly likely to happen' (SSI 1997: 3).

However, confusion continues to exist over the appropriateness of particular systems of restraint such as the 'Control and Restraint' system used in the Prison Service, whose officers trained staff at Aycliffe children's centre in County Durham in its use. The publicity given to allegations of physical abuse at Aycliffe was particularly unsettling for those working in children's institutions, as this was an institution that had acquired an international reputation for excellence and the 'bad apple' theory could consequently not be used as an explanation. The subsequent SSI report (1993) acknowledged that children had received injuries but did not attribute these to the 'Control and Restraint' system. Leadbetter (1995) notes that uncertainty exists as to which system of restraint includes which techniques and provides some useful guidelines on restraint systems.

The detailed definition of what is acceptable in terms of physical contact is a task left to local authorities. Lindsay (1995) stresses that policies on restraint need to be clear and specific so that staff will be confident in difficult situations, children will know what to expect and restraint techniques that are inappropriate and hidden do not develop. She also emphasises the dangers of staff not intervening when they need to act to protect a child. Restraint should be recognised as an extreme but inevitable form of control in institutions populated by adolescents who will be testing out a range of challenging behaviours and who will probably not have consented to their placement. In these circumstances, effective and acceptable methods of control that do not compromise individuals' dignity need to be available and clearly outlined.

Abuse from other residents

While the bullying and sexual violence experienced by children in boarding schools at the hands of their peers has been well-documented from Dickens onwards, it is only comparatively recently that such accounts would be defined as residential abuse. Chapter 2 of this book includes evidence of high levels of bullying in boarding schools and a study of four special boarding schools identified severe bullying as a problem for a minority of children (Grimshaw with Berridge 1994).

The NSPCC study (Westcott and Clément 1992), which included children abused in a range of institutions, identified 51 per cent of the main perpetrators of abuse as other children. All peer abusers were male and the main form of abuse suffered was sexual abuse. The extent to which children who have themselves been sexually abused may pose a risk to the safety of other children whom they live with is an issue that requires further clarification through research (National Children's Home 1992). However, children may enter residential settings with a known history of sexually abusing other children. Farmer and Pollock's study of sexually abused and abusing children in foster care and residential settings found that when new admissions were being considered, 'there was no mechanism to ensure that the child would be a good match with other children in the placement' (1998: 111). In this study, head teachers in residential schools were found to have more discretion than heads of homes who were often not able to refuse admissions. While only a small number of children included in this study (three out of a group of twenty-one) abused other children during the period they were in the residential settings, there were also examples of adolescent girls involving others in sexual behaviour that exposed them to risks.

Sinclair and Gibbs (1998) found that children in their sample who had been bullied in a previous setting were more likely to be bullied in their current institution. Past experience of bullying and sexual assault was associated with unhappiness, and current experience of bullying and sexual assault was even more strongly associated with being unhappy. This 'unhappiness' could be described more strongly as 'misery', with 39 per cent of Sinclair and Gibbs' sample having thought about killing themselves in the last month. Bullying has also been identified as a significant problem in secure accommodation (Howard League 1995). Barter (1997) argues that both sexual abuse and bullying in children's institutions frequently meet with responses of denial and minimisation from staff.

Bullying may also have a racial dimension. The respondents to the Who Cares? Trust survey were more likely to have experienced racist treatment from other children than they were from staff. Children in secure units were most likely to have experienced racism from their peers, but this was generally a problem for children in institutions rather than for children in foster care (Shaw 1998). While Black staff form a significant proportion of residential care staff in areas where there is a significant Black population, they remain at the lower levels of the staff hierarchy (Barn *et al.* 1997), and this is an issue that needs to be addressed in the light of racist behaviour between children.

Together with the evidence on bullying included in Chapter 2 of this book, these research studies portray a convincing picture of the abuse and accompanying distress that children in institutions experience at the hands of their peers. These studies offer little evidence of residential homes making use of the anti-bullying policies and strategies described by Mary MacLeod in the following chapter. Boarding schools have made more progress in this area in response to initiatives from the Department of Education (1994). The *Working Together* consultative document (Department of Health 1998b) promises central government guidance on effective anti-bullying strategies for residential childcare.

Gender and sexuality

As is the case with sexual abuse in the community, the vast majority of sexual abuse in institutions appears, from the inquiries, to involve male perpetrators. Where female staff are involved in physical abuse, it tends to be as collaborators rather than as instigators. Utting describes his experience of chairing the *People Like Us* review as 'a crash course in human (predominantly male) wickedness' (1997: 7), but the implications of this are not followed through other than to note the importance of gender issues (1997: 120). As is the case in all branches of social work, men are over-represented at the level of first-line management in residential child care (Balloch *et al.* 1995).

Wardhaugh and Wilding's (1993) influential analysis of institutional abuse identifies the balance of power and powerlessness as a significant factor in the 'corruption of care'. While staff in institutions may experience themselves as powerless in relation to the organisation, they are extremely powerful in relation to the children they care for. Wardhaugh and Wilding identify the combination of power and powerlessness as potentially dangerous and highlight gender inequalities as an additional complicating factor in the Pindown case. Berridge and Brodie's (1996) analysis of three inquiry reports identifies a 'macho' leadership or culture as common to all three regimes. Gender has an important role to play in structuring power relations within institutions. An individual man or small group of men charged with responsibility for managing a predominantly female workforce may feel extremely powerful within the confines of the institution, while experiencing himself or themselves as powerless in the managerial hierarchy. The gender balance and its impact on the distribution of power and authority within institutional settings merits more careful study and could be a factor used to inform staffing policies.

Throughout the inquiries and research studies reviewed here, expressions of male and female sexuality on the part of residents are identified as potentially threatening for staff. Farmer and Pollock (1998) comment on the stress experienced by male staff in the face of the highly sexualised behaviour of a few adolescent girls and note that residents' allegations of abuse by staff tended to result in the girls being handled punitively. Utting (1997) identifies the vulnerability of female staff to sexual harassment from male residents and staff (as does Brown in this volume). In settings dominated by adolescents, questions of how to identify, direct and communicate sexual feelings will inevitably loom large on the agenda. Aymer (1992) argues that women workers in children's homes are frequently asked to 'protect' male colleagues from 'dangerous' girls but are themselves expected to tolerate sexual harassment from male staff and boys alike. She also identifies race as a significant factor in determining how sexual activity among teenage girls is responded to by staff, with White staff more ready to tolerate activity that presents high risks of pregnancy for Black girls than they are for White.

Barter (1997) identifies the difficulties experienced by residential staff in tackling issues of sexuality and points out that it may be unrealistic to expect untrained staff to distinguish clearly between adolescent sexual experimentation and abuse. These difficulties are epitomised by the failure to manage teenage prostitution in some residential homes. Farmer and Pollock (1998) found that children involved in prostitution were one of the groups that were least likely to have their needs met in either foster or residential placements. They argue that friendship networks within the residential care system may serve to introduce children to prostitution and confirm them in that behaviour. They recommend the extension of child protection procedures to cover all children involved in prostitution and suggest that such a shift might serve to challenge the 'current rather passive attitude of residential staff' towards the issue (1998: 160). This shift in the Government's approach to child prostitution has already been announced (Department of Health 1998b) and can be expected to emerge as firm guidance when the new version of *Working Together* is published.

While there are real dangers in seeming to describe all institutions for children as characterised by high levels of violence and sexual aggression on the part of both staff and residents, it is evident that children's homes and special boarding schools contain many elements that can contribute to this picture. Such institutions house groups of sexually aware adolescents who are likely to be struggling with issues of peer group identity; some of these children have been abused in the past; the groups contain subgroups of more vulnerable children; and the majority of children will not have consented to their placement away from home. In the face of this scenario, the culture of the institution will be the main instrument for managing both staff and residents.

The institutional culture

Sinclair and Gibbs (1998) emphasise the significance of the culture of the individual establishment. They identify small size, a clear and stable role for the home, staff cohesion and agreement on common goals as key factors in developing a constructive culture. Similarly, in the Brown *et al.* (1998) study of nine children's homes the suggestion is that concordance between different sets of goals contributes to a healthy, positive staff culture. Both studies identified significant variations in culture between the homes studied.

The North Wales Tribunal has produced accounts from former managers of children's homes of cultures that now appear negative and damaging. The Tribunal has heard descriptions of how staff, jostling for position in the hierarchy, defined their place in the pecking order according to the degree to which they espoused a culture that one witness described as 'macho'. Features of such a culture included a game played at one home in the 1970s known as 'the war game', which involved staff and children charging at each other on the field. The disparity in size and strength meant, as the witness acknowledged, that the children invariably 'hit the deck first'. Witnesses justified the harshness of such regimes by describing the children as 'delinquents'.

It is not inconceivable that such a term would be used to describe children currently in institutions. Whilst inquiries and media coverage have talked in terms of 'children' and emphasised their vulnerability, Government reports in the 1990s stress that the majority of children in residential care are disruptive adolescents. This ambivalence has contributed to the low expectations from staff concerning the education of those in residential homes (Social Services Inspectorate and Office for Standards in Education 1995), and failures by a range of agencies to respond effectively to the needs of children who run away from residential care (Bridge Child Care Consultancy Service 1996). Wardhaugh and Wilding hark back to Goffman (1961) in identifying the definition of certain groups as 'less than full persons' (1993: 27) as another dynamic in the corruption of care. A positive culture in institutions will be informed as much by values and attitudes as it is by explicit goals and structures. Training might be expected to play a major role in developing values and positive attitudes, and also in identifying how values can be translated into practice. The discussion of the response to abuse in institutions will begin by considering the role of training.

Responding to abuse

Training

Throughout most of the 1990s, there was general agreement that a lack of qualifications and training among staff was one of the major problems besetting residential child care (Kahan 1994). Utting's (1997) reference to Sinclair and Gibb's (1998) failure to find an association between the quality of care provided in residential homes and the proportion of qualified staff has been interpreted as a major departure from this view (Ward and Preston-Shoot 1998). However, Sinclair and Gibbs (1998) suggest that their finding may reflect difficulties in staff groups where only a small proportion of staff are trained, as well as a dissonance between the content of training and the nature of the job. An increased interest in questioning the appropriateness of the Diploma in Social Work (DipSW) for residential child care staff has been another theme of the last decade, dating back to the Warner report (1992). Warner, and Lane (1994) after him, suggested that the European model of the 'social pedagogue' or *'educateur specialisé'* might offer a means of reconceptualising the role and training required for residential child care (see also Chapter 4). Milligan argues that the 'advice, guidance and assistance' (1998: 277) task of field social work is inappropriate for residential social work and that the two should be regarded as separate professions with different forms of training. A cautionary note is sounded by Crimmens who, while commenting that 'the UK appears to lag behind all its comparable European partners in training for residential child care' (1998: 312), found that there was no consideration of values in the social pedagogue training programme in the Netherlands.

While this debate has been developing, the Department of Health has proceeded with its Residential Child Care Initiative, announced in 1992, which aimed to increase the number of professionally qualified senior staff in children's homes. Additional funding was provided for nine DipSW programmes to recruit and train managers from residential care. Karban and Frost's (1998) analysis of the careers of graduates from three cohorts completing one of these programmes found that five out of thirty students had already left residential work, while another ten were contemplating leaving. While professional training was found to have been successful in developing students' confidence, former students also reported a sense of frustration when, back in the workplace, their criticisms of policy and resource matters met with little response. Utting (1997) notes the importance of employers valuing those who return to residential care work after professional training. However, such findings give weight to the arguments of those who advocate a distinct and separate training programme for residential care workers. Any such programme would need to be based on a new definition of the roles and tasks of the job, which position it more closely in relation to other services such as fostering and youth work. A realignment of this sort might offer a means of responding to Utting's (1997) fears that the residential child care sector is of insufficient size to support its own qualifying framework.

Interestingly, it is a requirement of approval by the Department of Education and Employment that the head of care in special residential schools has an appropriate qualification. Given that the number of officers-in-charge in local authority residential care homes with social work qualifications had risen to 83 per cent in 1995 (Utting 1997: 218), it would not seem unreasonable for the Government to introduce a similar requirement in all institutions for children within a fairly limited time-frame. However, it is clear that training for the heads of homes is insufficient on its own to transform a sector of staff whose self-esteem and specialised knowledge base are generally considered to be low. Training for basic-grade residential care staff has usually involved the National Vocational Qualification (NVQ) system, which focuses on identifying demonstrable competencies. Local authorities in England and Wales have introduced a Training Support Programme that aims to train residential care staff up to NVQ Level Three in Care. At the time of writing, the Department of Health has just announced a major initiative to improve the training level of all staff in children's homes. It is as yet unclear as to which model of training will be favoured for this programme, but it seems likely that a specified level of training will be a requirement of registration with the General Social Care Council (Brindle 1998).

Staffing

However, many of the staff at the centre of the inquiries into residential abuse possessed professional qualifications and there is increasing emphasis on regulating entry into the field of residential work with children. Utting (1997) recommends that the Warner report's (1992) proposals on issues such as job descriptions, person specifications, external advertising of posts, selection procedures and references should be extended to include educational institutions as well as children's homes. *People Like Us* also expresses concerns about delays in processing police checks and about the standard of proof required for names to be included on List 99, which identifies those who can be legally excluded from employment in educational settings. In addition, *People Like Us* notes that the Department of Health Consistency Index that includes names of those referred by the Social Services Department on the grounds that they are unsuitable to work with children (but carries no powers of exclusion from such work) is under-used by referrers. The SSI (1998) report, *Someone Else's Children*, also identifies confusion among social services staff as to when and if they should refer to the Index. In solving these problems, the Government's response to *People Like Us* includes the establishment of a new Criminal Records Agency that will facilitate easy access to both the Department of Education and the Department of Health lists for employers in social services and the voluntary sector (Secretary of State for Health 1998).

Staff vetting is also discussed in the *Working Together* consultation paper (Department of Health 1998b) that comments on the barriers to sharing information about those who are suspected but not convicted of offences against children, as well as noting the lack of guidance concerning what weight should be given to previous criminal convictions. However, the issue that perhaps raises most concern is the SSI (1998) finding that agencies supplying residential care staff were entrusted with responsibility for undertaking checks and that their performance in this area was often unmonitored. Given that in one authority inspected agencies supplied up to 45 per cent of residential care staff, this could represent a major weak link in recruitment procedures.

New guidelines based on the Department of Health Support Force for Children's Residential Care (1995) *Code of Practice for the Employment of Residential Workers* are soon to be issued (Secretary of State for Health 1998) and the long-awaited General Social Care Council will have a role in regulating membership of the workforce for residential care. Consideration may also be given to strengthening the position of whistle-blowers. Utting (1997) suggests the introduction of codes of conduct that would include a duty to report abuse and the nomination of a senior official who could initiate investigations in cases where complainants felt unable to approach their line manager.

The effect of this increased regulation and surveillance may well be to increase pressure on a workforce that already appears to be experiencing considerable stress. Whitaker *et al.*, in a study of staff groups in children's homes, found that staff were constantly wary of the possibility of allegations of abuse from the young people in their care. Residents threatened staff with their power to make allegations: 'I'll get you under the Act!' (1998: 224). Balloch *et al.* (1995), in a survey of the social services workforce, identified high levels of stress among managers of residential homes and found that both managers of residential homes and residential workers were more likely to have been physically attacked than other groups of staff. The need to monitor staff who work in institutions has to be carefully balanced against equal opportunities policies and the need for a workforce, already suffering from a poor self-image, to feel valued. Residential social work currently confronts the developments experienced by the nursing profession that, in response to the Clothier report (1994) on Beverley Allitt, tightened its entry requirements to a point that some have described as constituting oppressive practice (Manthorpe and Stanley 1999).

Management and inspection

At the level of the first line of management in children's homes, Sinclair and Gibbs (1998) identify the extent to which the head of home felt empowered as a key factor in securing positive outcomes. Empowerment emerges as more significant than autonomy and seems to involve managers understanding what is expected of them, being in agreement with those expectations and feeling confident enough to act creatively. Such an approach to management contrasts strongly with that of the SSI (1998), which focuses on monitoring standards; for instance, identifying a need to ensure that staff comply with departmental manuals.

It seems clear that the Department of Health's (1998a) *Quality Protects* programme will adopt the SSI audit model of setting standards and demanding evidence of progress towards them. The *Looking After Children (LAC)* materials are likely to be an important tool in this process in that they will facilitate the collection of data concerning children's needs, care plan objectives and progress towards them. Until now, LAC has been implemented on a voluntary basis; however, as 90 per cent of English local authorities have implemented the system (Jones *et al.* 1998), the use of the Assessment and Action Records for children who are looked after may become a requirement. As well as offering a combined audit and management tool, LAC provides the opportunity significantly to improve aspects of institutional care for children such as recording, planning and inter-agency work. It also offers a means of improving the status and practice of staff working with looked-after children. The dangers inherent in the system are that form-filling may take precedence over practice and impose heavy burdens on staff. Its relevance for use with children whose placements are short-term has also been questioned (Ballock 1998).

Many of the inquiry reports identify failings of senior management who turned a deaf ear to complaints, on the grounds that they had an investment in the continued existence of particular institutions or that they felt that they would be implicated in the failings of their staff. The introduction of an independent element into the complaints system may have reduced the possibility of complaints being discounted, but concerns remain that senior managers are reluctant to use disciplinary procedures in relation to those involved in institutional abuse (Utting 1997; SSI 1998). The report into 'The Trotter Affair' in Hackney (Barratt 1998) provides examples of failures to suspend a member of staff while he was under investigation.

The task of monitoring a large number of placements in small independent children's homes also makes demands on managers who frequently lack the resources required for such monitoring. The SSI Report (1995) into small unregistered children's homes found that fourteen authorities did not know that they were placing children in such accommodation. *Someone Else's Children* (SSI 1998) found that quality assurance checks on external providers varied considerably and identified both a lack of detailed standards that could be used to assess placements in the independent sector and a significant proportion of cases (26 per cent in one authority) where, as no social worker was allocated, monitoring of placements would inevitably be limited. Most worryingly, Berridge and Brodie (1998) report that the homes they studied in 1995 appeared to receive less external management support and monitoring than those they studied in 1985.

Under the Government's new proposals for the structure of inspection services, larger independent regional units will assume responsibility for inspections in both health and social services establishments (Department of Health 1998c). Utting (1997) sounds a warning note in pointing out that inspections of services for children may lose out in terms of priority and resources in larger units. Currently, residential children's homes and the residential provision of boarding schools are inspected by local authorities' Independent

Registration and Inspection Units; voluntary children's homes are inspected by the SSI; and the educational provision of boarding schools (including special schools) is inspected by OFSTED. There are difficulties in ensuring a free flow of information between the different inspectorates and Cawson (1997) identifies some of the inconsistencies between the different systems. The Burgner report (1996) recommended that all inspections be undertaken by a single authority and that small unregistered children's homes be brought within the regulatory framework. Utting (1997) notes the failure of 60 per cent of Social Services Inspection Units to meet the prescribed frequency of inspection, particularly in children's homes. Clearly, any new units with wider remits will need to be well resourced to undertake meaningful scrutiny of services.

Children's rights and representation

A children's rights perspective might be relevant in developing a response to the institutional abuse of children. The introductory chapter of *People Like Us* (Utting 1997) quotes the relevant articles of the UN Convention on the Rights of the Child that constitute the fullest statement of children's rights endorsed by the British Government. These articles have been used to underpin some of the campaigns mounted by groups such as Who Cares? and Article 12 that represent children in care.

In fact, as comparative studies of child protection systems have demonstrated (Hetherington *et al.* 1997), children's rights are given rather less prominence in the United Kingdom than in some other European states, with children being offered very little choice about which services *they* wish to receive and being allowed only a limited say in decisions that concern their welfare. Utting (1997) supports the British Association of Social Workers' (BASW) call for a set of legal rights applying to all children living away from home, and the recognition that children in institutions have a legal right to be free from assault might serve to shift perceptions of the status and moral worth of the child in institutional care.

Some structures already exist for the representation of children in institutions. Local authority complaints procedures require the involvement of independent persons and the Who Cares? Trust study (Shaw 1998) demonstrated that the majority of children were familiar with complaints procedures, with 73 per cent of those in children's homes saying that they knew how to make a complaint. The 1991 *Working Together* guidelines identify a need for an independent element to be included in the investigative team when allegations are made against an employee of the local authority managing the investigation, or when the local authority that looks after both the child and the abuser is the investigating authority. This process is explored in depth by Christine Barter in Chapter 3 of this book.

Children's rights and advocacy officers have been appointed to provide independent representation and support for children who are looked after; there were twenty-eight of these officers in post in 1995 (Willow 1996). The Children Act 1989 requires local authorities to appoint Independent Visitors for those children in out-of-home-care who have little or no contact with a parent. A survey of local authorities in 1996 found that only a third of local authorities in England and Wales were using Independent Visitors (Knight 1998). This study found that where volunteers were appointed as Independent Visitors for young disabled people they were able to act as advocates in review meetings as well as offering an experience of family life and a relationship with someone who was not in an official capacity. Utting (1997) recommends assessing the feasibility of extending the scheme but current funding mechanisms appear insecure. All children in secure accommodation receive a similar service from Independent Representatives.

The recent announcement by central government of funding for a national group (to be established under the auspices of First Key) that will represent children in care and care leavers (Department of Health 1998a) may constitute a shift towards recognising the centrality of a children's rights perspective in protecting children in institutions from abuse. However, with no underlying philosophy of children's rights to support current advocacy and representation services, they appear piecemeal and under-resourced. In the context of institutional care, children's rights are often perceived negatively so that 'within social work, children's rights has become almost synonymous with complaints' (Willow 1996: 69). At present, children's rights in the United Kingdom are supported by a limited legal and theoretical framework.

Children's institutions: a residual service?

The lack of theory informing work with children in institutions has in the past served to create a moral vacuum where abuse can prosper. Berridge and Brodie's 1998 study concludes that 'staff were not provided with a coherent explanation of children's problems and behaviour and a method or methods by which this could be addressed'

(1998: 153). The thinking justifying the continued use of residential homes and special boarding schools for children appears to be that for these groups of children there is no alternative. It might be argued that residential care for children has survived as a consequence of the failure to professionalise and divert funding into foster care. However, the case of Warwickshire, which closed all its children's homes in 1986 suggests that, while foster care is still conceived of as a non-professional service, the supply of foster carers is limited. The study of this closure identified an unproven possibility that more children were placed in special boarding schools (Cliffe with Berridge 1991).

It is perhaps in the residual nature of the service that alternative models for conceptualising residential care for children can be found. Many of the recent research studies into residential care explore the possibilities for integrating the work of residential homes with the care provided to children in families and foster homes. Berridge and Brodie identify an 'integrated model' (1998: 167) based on the role of specialist homes offering short breaks to disabled children. They argue that these homes conceptualised their task as 'a *service*' (1998: 169) for children and families, and demanded specialist skills and interprofessional work from staff. Sinclair and Gibbs (1998) also argue for more specialised homes and for breaking down the barriers between residential homes and other forms of provision. A positive role and philosophy might be identified for residential care as a specialist service offering support and respite to family-based forms of care and supported independent living schemes for care leavers. Freer movement of children between services might serve to avoid the development of bullying cultures in homes and offer children opportunities to disclose abuse at an early stage.

In the case of special boarding schools, such changes would require significant developments in the provision of education and care for disabled and disturbed children in the community. Whether independent boarding schools will survive in the face of the challenge mounted by independent day schools is a matter for parental choice and the state of the economy. In the immediate future many children will continue to live in institutions. If these children are to be protected from abuse, it is essential that they are seen as a group with clearly defined rights.

The recent policy response to the institutional abuse of children has been heavily shaped by inquiries and media coverage. The consequent focus on paedophiles represents a limited conception of institutional abuse and the picture needs to be broadened to include the study of power relations as mediated by age, gender, disability and race. While much hope is invested in systems of monitoring and setting targets, such systems run the risk of being meaningless paper exercises if institutional care for children lacks a purpose and a task that both staff and children can identify and perceive as having value.

References

Advisory Group on Video-recorded Evidence (1989) *Report of the Advisory Group on Video-recorded Evidence*, London: Home Office.

Aymer, C. (1992) 'Women in residential work: dilemmas and ambiguities', in M. Langan and L. Day (eds) *Women, Oppression and Social Work*, London: Routledge.

Balloch, S., Andrew, T., Ginn, J., McLean, J., Pahl, J. and Williams, J. (1995) *Working in the Social Services*, London: National Institute of Social Work.

Ballock, R. (1998) 'The use of LAC in child protection', *Children and Society* 12(3): 234–5.

Barn, R., Sinclair, R. and Ferdinand, D. (1997) *Acting on Principle: An Examination of Race and Ethnicity in Social Services Provision for Children and Families*, London: British Agencies for Adoption and Fostering.

Barratt, J. (1998) *The Report of the 1997 Inquiry into 'The Trotter Affair'*, London: London Borough of Hackney.

Barter, C. (1997) 'Who's to blame: conceptualising institutional abuse by children', *Early Child Development and Care* 133: 101–14.

Berridge, D. (1997) *Foster Care: A Research Review*, London: The Stationery Office.

Berridge, D. and Brodie, I. (1996) 'Residential child care in England and Wales: The inquiries and after', in M. Hill and J. Aldgate (eds) *Child Welfare Services: Developments in Law, Policy, Practice and Research*, London: Jessica Kingsley.

—— (1998) *Children's Homes Revisited*, London: Jessica Kingsley.

Brannan, C., Jones, R. and Murch, J. (1992) *Castle Hill Report Practice Guide*, Shrewsbury: Shropshire County Council.

Bridge Child Care Consultancy Service (1996) *In Care Contacts: The West Case, The Report of a Review of over 2,000 Files of Young Persons in Residential Care*, London: Bridge Child Care Consultancy.

Brindle, D. (1998) 'Children's home staff will have to be trained', *Guardian*, 23 October: 4.

Brown, E., Bullock, R., Hobson, C. and Little, M. (1998) *Making Residential Care Work: Structure and Culture in Children's Homes*, Aldershot: Ashgate Publishing.

Burgner, T. (1996) *The Regulation and Inspection of Social Services*, London: Department of Health and the Welsh Office.

Cawson, P. (1997) 'Who will guard the guards? Some questions about the models of inspection for residential settings with relevance to the protection of children from abuse by staff', *Early Child Development and Care* 133: 57–71.

Central Council for Training in Social Work and Department of Health Expert Group (1992) *Quality Standards for Residential Care*, London: Central Council for Training in Social Work.

Cliffe, D. with Berridge, D. (1991) *Closing Children's Homes: An End to Residential Childcare?*, London: National Children's Bureau.

Clothier, C. (1994) *The Allitt Inquiry: Independent Inquiry Relating to the Deaths and Injuries on the Children's Ward at Grantham and Kesteven General Hospital During the Period February to April 1991*, London: HMSO.

Crimmens, D. (1998) 'Training for residential child care workers in Europe: Comparing approaches in the Netherlands, Ireland and the United Kingdom', *Social Work Education* 17(3): 309–20.

Davies, N. (1998) 'The most secret crime – the epidemic in our midst', *Guardian*, 2 June: 5–6.

Department of Education (1994) *Bullying: Don't Suffer in Silence: An Anti-Bullying Pack for Schools*, London: HMSO.

Department of Health (1989) *The Care of Children: Principles and Practice in Regulations and Guidance*, London: HMSO.

—— (1991) *The Children Act 1989 Guidance and Regulations: Volume 4, Residential Care*, London: HMSO.

—— (1993) *Guidance on Permissible Forms of Control in Children's Residential Care*, London: Department of Health.

—— (1998a) *The Quality Protects Programme: Transforming Children's Services*, LAC (98) 28, London: Department of Health.

—— (1998b) *Working Together to Safeguard Children: New Government Proposals for Inter-Agency Co-operation, Consultation Paper*, London: Department of Health.

—— (1998c) *Modernising Social Services: Promoting Independence, Improving Protection, Raising Standards*, London: The Stationery Office.

Department of Health and Office for Standards in Education (1995) *The Education of Children Who Are Looked After by Local Authorities*, London: Department of Health and Office for Standards in Education.

Department of Health Support Force for Children's Residential Care (1995) *Code of Practice for the Employment of Residential Workers*, London: Department of Health.

Farmer, E. and Pollock, S. (1998) *Sexually Abused and Abusing Children in Substitute Care*, Chichester: Wiley.

Goffman, E. (1961) *Asylums*, Harmondsworth: Penguin.

Gooch, D. (1996) 'Home and away: The residential care, education and control of children in historical and political context', *Child and Family Social Work* 1: 19–32.

Grimshaw, R. with Berridge, D. (1994) *Educating Disruptive Children*, London: National Children's Bureau.

Hetherington, R., Cooper, A., Smith, P. and Wilford, G. (1997) *Protecting Children: Messages from Europe*, Lyme Regis: Russell House.

Home Office, Department of Health, Department of Education and Science, Welsh Office (1991) *Working Together under the Children Act 1989: A Guide to Arrangements for Inter-Agency Co-operation for the Protection of Children from Abuse*, London: HMSO.

Howard League (1995) *Banged Up, Beaten Up*, London: Howard League.

Jones, H., Clark, R., Kufeldt, K. and Norrman, M. (1998) 'Looking after children: Assessing outcomes in child care. The experience of implementation', *Children and Society* 12(3): 212–22.

Kahan, B. (1994) *Growing Up In Groups*, London: HMSO.

Karban, K. and Frost, N. (1998) 'Training for residential child care: Assessing the impact of the residential child care initiative', *Social Work Education* 17(3): 287–300.

Kirkwood, A. (1993) *The Leicestershire Inquiry 1992: The Report of an Inquiry into Aspects of the Management of Children's Homes in Leicestershire Between 1973 and 1986*, Leicester: Leicestershire County Council.

Knight, A. (1998) 'Independent visitors and disabled young people', *Findings*, January.

Lane, D. (1994) *An Independent Review of the Residential Child Care Initiative*, London: CCETSW.

Leadbetter (1995) 'Technical aspects of physical restraint', in The Centre for Residential Child Care, *Physical Restraint: Practice, Legal, Medical and Technical Considerations*, Practice Paper No. 2, June, Glasgow: The Centre for Residential Child Care.

Levy, A. and Kahan, B. (1991) *The Pindown Experience and the Protection of Children: The Report of the Staffordshire Child Care Inquiry 1990*, Stafford: Staffordshire County Council.

Lindsay, M. (1995) Chapter 2, in the Centre for Residential Child Care, *Physical Restraint: Practice, Legal, Medical and Technical Considerations*, Practice Paper No. 2, June, Glasgow: The Centre for Residential Child Care.

Local Government Management Board (1992) *The Quality of Care: Report of the Residential Staff's Inquiry (Chair Lady Howe)*, London: Local Government Management Board.

Loughran, F., Parker, R. and Gordon, D. (1992) *Children with Disabilities in Communal Establishments: A Further Analysis and Interpretation of the OPCS Investigation*, Bristol: Department of Social Policy and Social Planning, University of Bristol.

Manthorpe, J. and Stanley, N. (1999) 'Dilemmas in professional education: responding effectively to students with mental health problems', *Journal of Interprofessional Care*, forthcoming.

Milligan, I. (1998) 'Residential care is not social work', *Social Work Education* 17(3): 275–85.

Morris, J. (1995) *Gone Missing? A Research and Policy Review of Disabled Children Living Away from their Families*, London: Who Cares? Trust.

National Children's Home (1992) *The Report of the Committee of Enquiry into Children and Young People who Sexually Abuse Other Children*, London: National Children's Home.

Payne, M. (1997) *Modern Social Work Theory*, second edition, Basingstoke: Macmillan.

Secretary of State for Health (1998) *The Government's Response to the Children's Safeguards Review*, London: The Stationery Office. Cm 4105.

Shaw, C. (1998) *Remember My Messages: The Experiences and Views of 2000 Children in Public Care in the UK*, London: Who Cares? Trust.

Sinclair, I. and Gibbs, I. (1998) *Children's Homes: A Study in Diversity*, Chichester: Wiley.

Skinner, A. (1992) *Another Kind of Home: A Review of Residential Child Care*, Edinburgh: HMSO.

Social Services Inspectorate (1993) *'A Place Apart': An Investigation into the Handling and Outcomes of Serious Injuries to Children at Aycliffe Centre for Children, County Durham*, London: Department of Health.

—— (1995) *Small Unregistered Children's Homes*, London: Department of Health.

—— (1997) *The Control of Children in the Public Care: Interpretation of The Children Act 1989*, Chief Inspector Letter 20, February, CI(97)6, London: Department of Health.

—— (1998) *Someone Else's Children: Inspections of Planning and Decision Making for Children Looked After and the Safety of Children Looked After*, London: Department of Health.

Social Services Inspectorate and Office for Standards in Education (1995) *The Education of Children who are Looked After by Local Authorities*, London: HMSO.

Social Services Inspectorate, Wales and Social Information Systems (1991) *Accommodating Children: A Review of Children's Homes in Wales*, Cardiff: Welsh Office.

Utting, Sir W. (1991) *Children in the Public Care: A Review of Residential Child Care*, London: HMSO.

—— (1997) *People Like Us: The Report of the Review of the Safeguards for Children Living Away from Home*, London: The Stationery Office.

Ward, A. and Preston-Shoot, M. (1998) 'Editorial, special issue: Training and education for residential child care', *Social Work Education* 17(3): 269–74.

Wardhaugh, J. and Wilding, P. (1993) 'Towards an explanation of the corruption of care', *Critical Social Policy* 37: 4–31.

Warner, N. (1992) *Choosing with Care: The Report of the Committee of Inquiry into the Selection, Development and Management of Staff in Children's Homes*, London: HMSO.

Webster, R. (1998) *The Great Children's Home Panic*, London: Orwell Press.

Westcott, H. (1991a) *Institutional Abuse of Children: From Research to Policy, A Review*, London: NSPCC.

—— (1991b) 'The Abuse of Disabled Children: A Review of the Literature', *Child: Care Health and Development* 17: 243–58.

Westcott, H. and Cross, M. (1996) *This Far and No Further: Towards Ending the Abuse of Disabled Children*, Birmingham: Venture Press.

Whitaker, D., Archer, L. and Hicks, L. (1998) *Working in Children's Homes: Challenges and Complexities*, Chichester: Wiley.

Williams, G. and McCreadie, J. (1992) *Ty Mawr Community Home Inquiry*, Cwmbran: Gwent County Council.

Willow, C. (1996) *Children's Rights and Participation in Residential Care*, London: National Children's Bureau.

2 The abuse of children in institutional settings

Children's perspectives

Mary MacLeod

Outrage and anxiety have been the prevailing public responses to recent disclosures about the abuse of children in public care and boarding school. Public concern and press coverage have been instrumental in provoking Government action (Utting 1991; Warner 1992; Utting 1997; and the North Wales Inquiry, currently sitting). But if we are to get beyond outrage and anxiety to make things better for children, we have to listen to what they themselves have to say about who hurts them and what helps.

Calls from children to ChildLine (the UK national freephone helpline for children) about the impact of legal intervention are clear evidence that formal processes can silence children as much as abusers do (Keep 1996). Do we seriously think that inspectors visiting children's homes or schools could elicit from children complaints of abuse? Making residential settings safer for children cannot only be a matter of mechanisms, inspections, policing and child protection procedures, vital as these are. Children's testimonies direct us towards more comprehensive changes, involving both the culture of establishments and the quality of overall care provided.

This chapter describes what children living in children's homes and boarding schools have said to ChildLine about their experiences of sexual and physical assault. These are not completely similar groups of children. Children are generally in boarding school as a matter of parental and, often, child choice – a very different matter from those living in children's homes as a result of family disruption, abuse, maltreatment, or on a legal order, sometimes against their own or their family's wishes (see Chapter 1 of this volume). But important aspects of their experience are the same: such children do not have their own family to return to and turn to at night; they are reliant on fellow residents for support; opportunities exist for fellow residents and staff to assault them; getting help is complicated; access to independent adults is not easy; and high-profile exposés of assaults suggest that sex offenders form networks to target such children.

My aim is to place the abuse of children in residential settings in the context of their other possible concerns about where they live. Open systems are less corruptible than closed ones. Research shows that adults who exploit children sexually target children who are separate from their usual family network and who are unhappy, lonely, isolated or feel unwanted. Those children with previous histories of sexual or physical assault, or of behaviour difficulties, or those with disabilities affecting communication will also be targeted (Conte 1990; Dobash *et al.* 1993; Colton and Vanstone 1996). This is a matter of strategy and opportunity: the very depth of the need to feel wanted, alongside isolation from steady support, can make children easier prey.

Safeguarding children, then, requires attention to the entire environment of children living away from home. And here inspection and regulation have a clear, indispensable role.

The research evidence

I draw on evidence from three ChildLine studies (La Fontaine and Morris 1991; Lees *et al.* 1994; MacLeod 1997) examining calls from over 5,000 children in the United Kingdom living away from home, and call statistics from 1997–8. The calls were made either to the ChildLine 0800 1111 main service (open twenty-four hours a day, every day) or to two special lines: one for children in boarding schools (a six-month long project in 1991) and the other for children in care (from 1992 to the present, open four hours each day). Child callers refer to themselves as 'in care' and never 'looked after'; 'in care' and 'living away from home' are the phrases used in this chapter to describe their position.

ChildLine's data is held in two forms: a written record completed immediately after the conversation with the child, and a computer record of details with a summary of the conversation with the child, input from the written record by administrative staff. The computer-held data allows statistical and text analysis on the very large numbers of child callers. However, since the counselling conversation is conducted to serve the child rather than research, the information offered is not uniform, and there are many 'no data' entries.

Despite the Department of Health and the Department for Education and Employment guidance to homes and schools about access to phonelines, we cannot be certain that all children who wish to phone are free to do so; and we know for sure that all who wish to cannot get through to ChildLine because the phones are so busy (MacLeod 1996a). Thus, calls to the helpline cannot tell us about the prevalence of abuse in residential settings, only about the instances described to us by individual children and the commonality and differences in their experiences. Though the sample is not representative, here we have the authentic voices of children telling it like it is, for them.

In residential care

'I just want to feel wanted.' This is how one 14-year-old girl summed up her own desire and that of many children in public care – a basic human need, yet unattainable for many. In all, 1,168 girls and 446 boys called ChildLine from care in the year up to 31 March 1996, of whom 1,130 were living in residential units. Children in residential care are at least eight times more likely to call than children living at home. They mainly call about problems in care (20 per cent): decision making; sanctions; unhappiness with placement, keyworker or social worker; feeling bad about being in care; contact and loss; sexual and physical abuse at home and in care (20 per cent); bullying and violence in care (9 per cent); and running away (11 per cent).

Most calls are from 11 to 15 year olds, with fewer younger children calling than on our general service (under 4 per cent, compared with 9.5 per cent). It is not possible to provide a reliable ethnic breakdown from ChildLine data because all children do not provide this information. Where children do, it is noted. Two per cent of child callers to the Children in Care Line said they were Black or from an ethnic minority group, and less than 1 per cent calling 0800 1111 did so.

Children in public care are among the most troubled, isolated, unhappy children calling ChildLine, conveying a picture of family dislocation and formidable loss, of abuse, transient care arrangements and frequent moves. A constant theme in their conversations has been their sense of abandonment, unimportance and low self-esteem; another, a deep sense of confusion about why events had turned out as they had – even uncertainty about the reasons for their admission to care, or why things that they really wanted could not happen.

> Alex, 12, called because he had had a review that day and the social workers discussed having his sisters adopted but did not discuss his future. He and his two sisters had lived with his foster parents for nearly 18 months after being sexually abused by his mother's boyfriend. He did not want to be separated from his

sisters; he wanted to stay with the foster parents where they were all happy. He said the foster parents wanted this too but the social worker didn't listen. He wanted to know whether he could do anything about this.

Children call ChildLine about what is wrong rather than what is right. Their experiences need to be read in the context of other studies and in the knowledge that for some children entry into care is a great relief. The Who Cares? Trust study found that 67 per cent of their respondents from residential care described themselves as happy, and that 47 per cent said there was always someone they could talk to if they felt sad, lonely, worried or depressed (Shaw 1998). The study found that 8 per cent of girl respondents and 15 per cent of boy respondents described coming into care as 'great'; and 12 per cent said the best thing about being in care was having someone who cares. But these proportions also convey a dismal implication: what of the others?

ChildLine callers described periods of acute emotional turmoil, episodes of rage against themselves or others, drug use, behaviour problems, long-standing relationship difficulties with families and with carers, and times of deep depression marked by despair and suicidal feelings. They often said that they could not confide their concerns to their carers and social workers because they did not see them; or they felt that they were not taken seriously, that everyone would find out, or that the adults did not have the time for them.

A very few callers talked about seeing their social workers every week – the honourable exceptions. There was little sense of children having their workers available on the telephone – surely easy to arrange – or of people outside the 'care frame' being emotionally available to them. Mainly they, like their counterparts living at home (Keep 1996), confided in and relied on their friends for support and comfort; but these friendships were often disrupted by moves.

Mandy, 15, called because she was cutting herself after hearing that her friend had gone away for a few days. She was terrified she wouldn't come back. 'My life is a mess. ... My brother committed suicide in June. ... I've got a new boyfriend and he's pushing me to have sex. ... Mum came to see me last week for the first time since my brother died ... we ended up fighting and she hit me in the face. ... I just can't talk to the staff ... Jacky is the only friend I have ... the only one I can talk to ... '

The support that friends provide can be built upon. Effort spent on keeping young people in touch with their friends, and in establishing peer support and mentoring schemes, uses the relationships children often trust the most and their own considerable resources.

Though these are children who have known terrible inconsistency and loss, their lives in care are highly disrupted by moves. Of 840 child callers to ChildLine's special line for children in care who talked about their moves, one in four had moved more than four times, and one in ten said 'many' or more than ten. These are shameful statistics.

Some youngsters have to move for purely financial reasons, at short notice, forced to uproot themselves just as they are settling down with new relationships, getting close to a care worker or other children. They imply that they have no say in decisions made about them, confirming their view of themselves as negligible and unwanted.

> Ruth, 15, called to ask if she could complain about social services. She is now in a children's home where she is happy but in the past she was moved around a lot. 'I want to complain about neglect. ... I was just shoved around ... every time I behaved badly I was just moved on.' Ruth said that her social worker supported her in making a complaint; but that he was nervous he would lose his job if he did.

When young people, like Ruth, demonstrate their resilience and begin to take an active interest in organising their own lives, rejecting the plans made for them, they can be seen as 'making trouble'. Instead, the drive they have found requires encouragement. They may well not always be right in their objective, but the will and readiness to try are likely to be their greatest allies in the struggle to overcome the difficulties life has dealt them. But it is hard for care staff and social workers within local authorities to support resistance against the agency that employs them, highlighting the necessity of access to independent sources of help.

In boarding school

Calls by almost 1,300 children and young people, calling from boarding school, have been reviewed by ChildLine in two studies (La Fontaine and Morris 1991; MacLeod 1997). Overall, there was not the same multitude of problems, nor transience of place and relationship: these callers had a strong sense of home and place. Yet young people in the sample did convey a marked sense of loneliness, isolation and homesickness. When things went wrong, they felt on their own. The proportion of youngsters talking about mental health problems and suicidal feelings far outstripped those calling ChildLine generally (10 per cent, compared with 4 per cent on the national service).

The profile of problems was markedly different to general calls to ChildLine. Eighteen per cent identified school problems (compared with 2 per cent of our whole constituency for the same year); 16 per cent bullying (compared with 12 per cent); 6 per cent sexual abuse (compared with 10 per cent) and 5 per cent physical abuse (compared with 9 per cent). The reasons given for feelings of unhappiness at school included problems with school-work, exams and/or sporting activities. However, the main areas of concern mentioned were: home-sickness and missing parents; dislike of and unhappiness in school; loneliness and having no friends; and difficulties over school discipline. Children usually felt unable to tell their parents, fearing that their feelings would be dismissed or that their parents would be disappointed – especially when parents were investing so much money in their education.

Bullying in residential homes and schools

Yvonne, 13, described being bullied in her children's home. She had thought about running away. She was in care because a family friend abused her and her mum did not believe her. A review was coming up and she was scared of being sent home. She wanted to stay in care despite the bullying.

Jenny, 15, was in care in a residential school. The previous month she had been violently kicked and hospitalised by another resident. She described the bullying in the school as constant and said it was ignored by staff. She had complained to her social worker but nothing was done. She felt her social worker always deferred to the school staff.

Bullying is a child protection concern, not only because of bullying behaviour but also because the impact on children with no home refuge can be devastating – suicide and running away are serious risks. A third of runaway children in the earlier ChildLine study were attempting to escape bullying (Lees *et al.* 1994).

Bullying was the overriding difficulty of 16 per cent of those in boarding school and 9 per cent of those in children's homes. Few callers felt that they could get help with the bullying in either setting. They were very fearful of the consequences of telling because they had no confidence that they could be properly protected if they did tell. Sometimes the picture was of institutionalised bullying, sometimes of a complete breakdown of staff control, and sometimes of invidious, secretive types of harassment – extremely difficult for adults to observe, far less to intervene and stop.

In some homes bullying was rife, with staff seemingly unable to protect children.

> 'I'm frightened in the home I'm in ... I just feel desperate ... I want to kill myself.' Toni, 14, said the staff had no control. She described eight residents who were very aggressive and intimidating. The week before she had come, a child had been stabbed. The home was private ' ... but social services pay for me to be there. My social worker thinks I'm exaggerating ... I just want to get away from here.'

> Louise, 13, had been in her present children's home for six months. She had been in care for three years and had moved a number of times. In her present home she was being repeatedly assaulted by fellow residents. 'Yesterday they punched and kicked me ... the staff try to help ... but they can't stop them ... they always get me in the end. ... I've taken overdoses ... I can't go on ... I'm thinking of running away.'

Though the violence involved in these instances is alarming, verbal bullying has a pernicious effect on children, particularly when there is no escape night or day: 'I hear them all the time; they go on and on. I can't get their voices out of my head.'

Many of the verbal taunts referred to the very experiences with which children were struggling to cope. It was not unusual for girls to be called 'a slag' when it emerged that they had been abused. Nor was it unusual for this to precipitate a further assault. Others, like Paul below, were taunted about their looks or sexuality. Yet others faced racist bullying. ChildLine research suggests that single Black children in homes or schools (or one of few other Black or ethnic minority children) require particular vigilance by staff so that early signs of exclusion or bullying can be picked up and dealt with (MacLeod 1996b).

Joanne, a 10-year-old Black girl at boarding school, was being relentlessly bullied by a girl in her class, who called her racist names. Joanne had one friend who would stick up for her but it was getting her down and she was not doing well in class. She felt she would be too embarrassed to tell her mum whom she was missing very badly.

Anita, 13, being bullied in school, said, 'Mum and Dad didn't take it seriously. ... I decided I didn't want to live ... I took paracetamol ... they made me sick ... I'm stabbing myself with scissors ...'

Paul, 12, was being bullied verbally and physically. 'They call me fat and gay and a girl.' His father was now visiting him at school less and that was really upsetting. He was bingeing on food and then making himself sick.

Such levels of fear, intimidation and violence are wholly unacceptable, as is adult unwillingness or reluctance to act. Though boarding schools have long been concerned about bullying, it is only recently that the significance of the problem of bullying in care has been recognised (Utting 1997).

Tried and proven anti-bullying strategies could be used to change residential cultures and support individual children. 'Whole-school' approaches, school-based violence prevention programmes, and child assault prevention schemes (Suderman *et al.* 1993), could be reworked as 'whole institution' strategies (Tattum and Herbert 1993; Department of Education 1994; Sharp and Smith 1994; Smith and Sharp 1994; MacLeod and Morris 1996). Drama, role play, video and discussion groups can engage young people in general discussion and help them to practise self-help strategies. Group approaches, for example the 'no-blame' approach, 'quality circles', and the 'method of common concern' (Sharp and Smith 1994; MacLeod and Morris 1996) can be used to tackle group bullying. Peer counselling, mentoring and mediation schemes (Cowie 1995) have many applications as well as supporting individual children. They have been shown to involve increased self-esteem for the counsellors, an outcome worth pursuing in itself (Cowie 1995).

Each residential setting should have a senior member of staff delegated to develop strategy and train staff to ensure that dealing with bullying is a priority. Homes and schools could begin with anonymous questionnaires to map the problem and engage young people in providing solutions. Thus, the experience of developing anti-bullying strategies could be an instrument in promoting good pastoral care in homes, and so contributing to a more open, and thus safer, culture.

Sexual and physical assault in schools and homes

There are now fewer reports of assault from children in residential settings than there were earlier in ChildLine's lifetime (MacLeod 1997). Most children in institutional settings now call about sexual and physical abuse by family members rather than care staff or teachers; abuse by other children is also significant and largely undetected. This underlines the importance of a strategy that takes account of the prevalence of familial abuse and abuse by other children, as well as the dangers of sex offenders in the wider community.

In any process of counting incidences of abuse, the numbers depend on definition, and definitions vary from child to child and between children and adults. This is a constant problem in research on child abuse (Kelly *et al.* 1991; Dartington Social Research Unit 1995; MacLeod 1996a). Calls here were defined as abuse when the child defined them as such; but this involves an underestimate, since young people describe quite serious assaults as bullying, and sexual assaults by peers and boyfriends are under-reported.

Tables 2.1 and 2.2 show the numbers and proportions of children in residential care and boarding school complaining about assault in the various studies reported here; as well as statistics from 1997–8. The 1994 study on children in care did not give a breakdown on the perpetrators of physical abuse; so it is not possible to say how many of the twelve children complaining about physical abuse as a main problem were assaulted by care workers, but extrapolating from the breakdown in other samples, it is likely to be less than half.

Table 2.1 Assaults in residential care by staff

Number	1992 sample N: 278				1995–6 sample N: 1,130				1997–8 sample N: 701			
	Sexual abuse		Physical abuse		Sexual abuse		Physical abuse		Sexual abuse		Physical abuse	
Perpetrators	no.	%	no.	%	no.	%	no.	%	no.	%	no.	%
Staff	8	2.8	c.5	c.1.8	20	1.7	19	1.8	11	1.6	10	1.4

Table 2.2 Assaults in boarding schools

Number	1992 sample N: 1,000				1995–6 sample N: 289			
	Sexual abuse		Physical abuse		Sexual abuse		Physical abuse	
Perpe-trators	no.	%	no.	%	no.	%	no.	%
Staff	110	11	38	3.8	8	2.8	7	2.4
Children	27	2.7	6	0.6	4	1.4	12	4.2
Parents	18	1.8	12	1.2	11	3.8	11	3.8

In the context of the considerable public anxiety about institutional abuse of children, it is striking that the proportion and numbers of complaints on the helpline have fallen (reflecting the position on the national service where proportions have also fallen). We can only hope it means that the public awareness and increased openness about sexual assaults are having an impact. But it may be no more than a reflection of either ChildLine's life-span – as those children who had nowhere to go previously created a peak of calls about abuse early on in the helpline's life – or differences in the accessibility and promotion of the service.

Though there has been a reduction in reports of abuse by teachers from children in boarding school, they still seem to be more at risk of abuse from teachers than those in day school (MacLeod 1997). In 1995–6, ChildLine was almost fifty times more likely to hear about physical assaults and nine times more likely to hear of sexual assaults by teachers from children in boarding school. Complaints about sexual assaults by fellow students were also more likely (four times so).

It was difficult to establish with certainty if an abuser was assaulting children other than the caller since the child might not have known. One record from the 1995–6 boarding-school sample of 289 gave rise to concern that the abuse suffered might be part of a regime of violence; three records referred to teachers who were believed to have abused other children, as did several from the care sample.

Mark called to say he thought allegations being made about staff at his home must be true because they played a game called 'hairy monsters' that involved exposing themselves. 'One of the staff bullied me into doing things [and] … pressured me into going on nature walks to do things.' The man concerned was now suspended and Mark was wondering if he should tell what happened to him, but he felt ashamed.

None of the children complaining about abuse found it easy to get help. Telling was only the first hurdle; being taken seriously when they told was equally challenging; and dealing with the furore following disclosure was yet another enormous struggle. Most preferred not to speak.

Sexual assaults in residential homes

Almost all of the young people in care complaining about assaults had also been abused in the past:

> Sarah was calling from the children's home where she has lived since she was abused by her dad. 'I just started to trust people again and now I'm being abused again by someone who works here.' Sarah had attempted suicide that week.

> Leanne, 13, described one of the care staff coming into her room at night and touching her. She was in care because of sexual abuse by her father.

Fathers and stepfathers remained the most likely assailants of children sexually assaulted while in care, commonly a continuation of abuse that brought about their reception into care. Children in these situations, unsurprisingly, feel there is nothing to be done. Young people have described resisting a push for them to return home but being unable to tell their social worker or care worker that the abuse was continuing. Staff need to be alive to the possibility of a continuation of abuse, and to the difficulty children have in saying so.

Over 11 per cent (249) of the children in residential care who rang ChildLine in 1995–6 had run away. They are a highly vulnerable group of youngsters, easy prey for exploitative adults, and prime targets for those who appear to offer care and loving – as the Bridge report into runaway children in Gloucestershire, bears out (Bridge Child Care Consultancy Service 1996). Those who had run away (like those feeling suicidal) frequently described sexual or physical assaults, or bullying as the reason.

If children are simply returned to their care placements with no questions asked, they are likely to run again. But breaking through the barrier of mistrust and fear is not easy. Staff frustration at repeat runaways can spill over into an uncaring response, where, for example, the fact that a runaway is also only a 12-year-old child no longer has an impact.

Young troubled people on the streets can be endangered whether they are 'on the run' or not. And if they are assaulted, then stereotyped ideas about them can lead to their receiving an unequal, prejudiced response.

> Carla, 15, called ChildLine to ask for help following a serious sexual assault by a police officer. It took the ChildLine counsellor talking directly to the police and indicating that there was likely to be forensic evidence to begin the process of investigation. Once begun, it was conducted in exemplary fashion.

All of the assailants in the 1995–6 sample were male, whether resident or staff member. The prevalence of assaults by fellow residents – responsible for more than half of assaults in care (MacLeod 1997) – argues for an end to placing children who have been victimised with those who have abused, and the urgency of therapy for both. The predicament of young male victims who are also perpetrators is highlighted in Callum's story:

> Callum came to the attention of social services following his sexual assault on his stepsister; only then did it emerge that he himself had been assaulted by his stepfather over many years. Though he was a victim, he was only perceived as an abuser and neither his family nor his local authority wanted to give him a home. Eventually, a therapeutic placement was found but not before he had made a serious suicide attempt. Throughout this period and his therapeutic placement, his most stable contact was a ChildLine counsellor.

Children in residential care were much more likely to have been sexually assaulted prior to the assault by a member of staff than children in boarding school. They were also more likely to have additional difficulties that, arguably, would make it harder for them to recover; and more likely to respond in ways that created even more risk of continuing assault, like running away. They were less likely (from those talking to ChildLine, at any rate) to ask for help than those from boarding school. It is as if they felt that their quota of belief had been used up; or that they had been through the 'child protection' mill before, finding it ineffective and traumatic; or that they felt nothing could be done; or it was just that they expected and were resigned to such experiences.

Perhaps worst of all was the feeling of self-blame, worsened and deepened by further assaults, the abusers' rationalisations, sexual misuse by boyfriends, and disbelieving responses. Summaries like this, in plotting the course of likely effects of assault, can appear to be prescribing an inevitable downward spiral. Such accounts can, in turn, lead professionals into anticipating poor outcomes. The prevailing discourse can blunt the child or young person's resistance and the professional's reluctance to accept such an outcome, and thus contribute to a dynamic that produces what it attempts to avoid.

It is invidious to describe one group's plight as more serious than another's. Children in boarding school share with those in care vulnerability to assault, isolation from sources of help, and the trauma where abuse occurs. Both groups need responsible adults to act to protect them. Those in boarding school seemed marginally readier to trust a teacher with what had happened, but that did not always secure protection.

Sexual assaults in boarding schools

> 'The head teacher has been "feeling me" in bed.' The boy had heard that this had happened before and his senior master (whom he had evidently told) was sympathetic; but, 'I'm going to be in a lesson with him [the head teacher] tomorrow and I'm scared.'

> Paul, 15, was sometimes touched sexually by a teacher in the book cupboard, he has told his form teacher who ' … is going to help the other teacher to stop it'.

Yet other teachers appear to exploit children's vulnerability:

> Gordon's teacher was kind and put his arm around him when he was homesick and upset, but now is touching him, coming into his room. Gordon can't tell his parents or the school; he rang because he did not want to return to school.

> Another boy told of receiving verbal advances from a male teacher. He was frightened and felt threatened and unable to

handle the situation, but felt he could not tell anyone because the teacher might lose his job.

Of the four youngsters complaining about sexual assaults by fellow pupils, two described rapes.

> A girl had been raped by an older boy; she had told her mother and the police were now involved. She was very anxious about what would happen next and about going to court.

> A teenage boy described being gang-raped by four older boys; he was bruised and bleeding and had told matron that he had a stomach ache. He was not prepared to tell anyone about it because the boys said they would do it again if he did. He had joined the school from prep school that year and liked it until now. This boy was in shock and very frightened. The counsellor was at pains to urge him to confide in someone and let him know there was very likely to be medical evidence and that he would be believed. He resolutely refused to give any identifying information but did say he would think seriously about telling.

This incident bears hallmarks of institutionalised abuse. It raises questions about the prevalence of such attacks in the school and if the young perpetrators had themselves been introduced to violent sexual assault as victims of older boys or teachers.

It was extremely perturbing to find that telling an adult did not necessarily stop the abuse. The teachers approached seemed unwilling or unable to act on the information they had received. Children described a silence following their complaint, or not being told what the teacher planned to do, if he had done it, and what the outcome would be.

Physical assaults in residential homes and boarding schools

Most complaints about physical assault from children living away from home were about their parents or foster parents – as with sexual assaults. Youngsters differentiated between physical assaults and discipline, though the borderline seemed thin to this reader: one youngster described being caned regularly at school and beaten at home – for minor lapses of behaviour. Yet others described violence as institutional:

> Jack, 13, rang about an initiation rite involving boys being put in messy baths and having their heads pushed down the toilet – all the boys in his year (the first) were terrified but could do nothing about what was happening.

Physical assaults on older children are not generally life-threatening, so they tend not to be taken as seriously as sexual assaults. Much of the abuse reported here occurred in the context of children's behaviour when they were being, or were seen to be, disruptive or 'out of control'. Staff attempting to restrain or discipline them 'lost it' or lost all sense of proportion.

> Rosie, 15, called from a secure unit. She described food being withheld, being forcibly restrained and hit, and locked in her room for long periods of time. She wanted help to contact her social worker.

> Greg, 16, was supposed only to be accommodated for three months, but he had been in the home for six months now and didn't know when he would get home. He said he kept being restrained on the floor and hit. He had seen his social worker on the day he called and told her about it; but he thought she might think he was making it up because she knew he didn't want to stay.

Other children described being picked on by a staff member, though this was the pattern in assaults committed by other children rather than those by care staff. However, when a young person did feel 'picked on', it could be hard to convince staff.

> Jason said he was picked on all the time by one care worker who had grabbed him that night and torn his jumper. He tries to tell the other staff but nothing happens.

Staff are likely to find it extremely hard to pick each other up on unfair treatment. It requires effective group supervision to make this routine practice even in the most experienced staff groups.

Young people were disarmingly frank about the outbursts of feeling and frustration that precipitated these crises. Often, they felt out of control and wanted to talk about how this might be stopped. There was little evidence from children in residential care (unlike boarding school) of creative, leisure and sports pursuits being available, though one boy explicitly described how he had taken up football to relieve the tension brought about by memories of violent sexual abuse by his step-father. Therapy or counselling were infrequently mentioned. The overriding impression was of a warehousing process where boredom prevailed; though, of course, ChildLine does not hear the good news about care.

Few remedies or options seem to the children to be available. There is a level of acceptance of physical violence affecting children themselves, unsurprising in a country where 90 per cent of children are hit by their parents (Smith *et al.* 1995), and one-in-four primary-school children and one-in-ten secondary-school children suffer bullying each term (Smith and Sharp 1994), around half of which is physical (MacLeod and Morris 1996).

Children and young people do not find it easy to complain, whether or not they know about the existing complaints procedures. They tend to formulate what has happened as a problem rather than a complaint. Fear of repercussions, of getting staff into trouble, of being moved or having everything taken out of their hands are commonly cited as the reasons children prefer not to speak. These are often children who have been through the gamut of legal processes – often finding the process excluding, unjust and abusive (Keep 1996). In addition, complaints processes are, at best, bureaucratic and take time; young people, and especially younger children, give up or cannot contemplate initiating a complaint without independent advocates to support them.

Therapy and pastoral care

Perhaps the most dispiriting feature of the young people's lives in residential care was the absence of attention to their emotional recovery. This was something children themselves recognised and deeply regretted:

> 'The staff just don't have time for me. ... I don't like to ask them to come and talk ... '

> 'I've been depressed lately ... I've run away a few times ... I feel everyone has turned against me. ... ' Jake, 15, had been returned to his residential home following a suicide attempt. He described the Head immediately turning on him and accusing him of stealing. He was not seeing anyone to talk about his feelings of despair.

When support was available to young people, they valued it:

'She was really good. She gave you good advice and I felt there was someone on my side who was willing to help me and, you know, show me the right directions.' A 16-year-old talking about her previous social worker.

Children actively wanted help to reflect on and come to terms with what had happened to them. They wanted to be able to discuss the complexities of their family relationships and the circumstances that brought them into care – many were still unclear about why this had happened. But they were deeply hesitant about trusting themselves to this endeavour, especially when they felt that their personal histories and feelings were so public within the care system, and when they have to live alongside those from whom they are expected to receive help.

'It's a lovely home ... the people are really nice ... but I'm just not getting on with them ... I'm angry all the time. ... I think it's because I've been thinking about my mum ... I have had arguments with two staff ... I feel upset and angry whenever anyone mentions Mum in any way.' Chantelle, 11, was in care because ' ... Dad did something to me and Mum. ... I don't want to talk about it ... it's too painful.'

The extent of loss, disruption, rejection, inconsistency and abuse suffered by many of these youngsters defies belief; it should galvanise adults into action to help them recover. Offering therapeutic help is not some luxury far too costly to entertain seriously. If we want to reduce their vulnerability to assault from predatory adults and from each other, it is essential. Children's use of services that they access themselves has overturned many of the conventions of orthodox counselling and therapy (Cowie 1995; Epstein 1995 and 1996; Barter *et al.* 1996; MacLeod 1996a); we need to have a rich and varied menu from which young people themselves can choose. So, as this chapter argues, a great deal can be accomplished using the resources of children themselves – allowing them to be the experts on their own lives.

Getting help

Though the children reported here do not convey an impression of experiencing endemic sexual violence, many felt unable to ask for help. Even more perturbing was the reluctance of those they confided in to act according to the guidance laid down. Children in care were more likely than those in boarding school to describe not being taken seriously by adults to whom they reported abuse. The adults, seemingly, assumed they were complaining in order to manipulate or bring about a change in their placement.

> 'I told my social worker; but she thinks I'm making it up to get out of here.' A 15-year-old in a secure unit.

Children in boarding school did not report disbelief, simply inaction. In three out of the eight examples from boarding school, the teacher's proclivities were apparently common knowledge and tolerated. One prosecution and conviction emerged from these complaints because a teacher bravely took action on learning about the abuse (a call to ChildLine had been overheard). Even so, the court process was traumatic for the child who had serious second thoughts about giving evidence.

Callers had three major anxieties: that they would not be taken seriously and believed; that matters would get worse for them rather than better – they would get into trouble, the abuse would continue, they would be moved; and that matters would immediately be taken out of their control. Exactly the same concerns were expressed by children abused by fellow residents. In consequence, children tolerated abuse and were driven to risky solutions that often endangered them further.

Although we are aware that *Working Together* (Home Office *et al.* 1991), the official guidance on child protection to professionals in all agencies, is being rewritten, policy as it now stands assumes that investigation is the inevitable consequence of a child describing abuse. What children have to say shows that this often means moving too fast and too definitively for them. In such a process there are only two choices for children: to 'put up with' the abuse or the investigation – put up or shut up. Children are usually asking for the abuse to stop and for emotional support; they are unprepared for the course that can follow a request for help to achieve this. They require help in anticipating the quality and range of evidence required so that they are armed with something apart from their word in a process where their word counts for very little.

Creating child protection procedures that do not, inadvertently, collude in silencing children is difficult. It cannot be done without allowing some element of discretion to those in whom children confide. This is a thorny dilemma: if discretion is increased, how will organisations and individuals cope with the wave of public opprobrium when things go wrong, as they inevitably will? Can professional discretion be trusted in the absence of quality training? Will increased discretion just lead to a 'dumbing down' of complaints?

If discretion is too risky to encourage, then the best hope comes from ensuring that each child and young person has access to (and knows they have access to) their families (wherever possible) and to independent sources of help; and that peer support is actively encouraged (since children are most likely to confide in friends). Just as parents will talk in a low key way to their child about the kinds of things that can hurt them and what to do when they are in trouble, so too should care staff and teachers have that kind of conversation with children in their care. However good the procedures are, if children do not get the message that they will be listened to and taken seriously, they are simply not going to be in any position to risk saying anything. If there is one lesson to be learned from all the inquiries into failures to protect children or prevent abuse, it is that children will not shout until they make themselves heard; rather they require patient encouragement and adults available to them, who are neither blind to the possibility of abuse, nor afraid to hear it.

Regimes of abuse prosper because people deny, minimise or rationalise what is happening: 'it is just touching' or 'it will not really do any harm'. Adults appear to consider it more serious for a fellow adult to face the ignominy of being found responsible for sexual misconduct, than for a child to be assaulted. Or they cannot face the fuss and trauma involved in taking such matters up. Few adults seem brave enough to do so if the alleged offender is in authority over them. 'Whistle-blowing' has never been easy. Legal protection for whistle-blowers is now greater than it was; many organisations have already taken steps to highlight staff's responsibility to draw wrongdoing to the attention of management, but cultures have to change as well as the legal framework.

The head is usually the dominant influence on the culture of homes and schools. Their leadership and style should be regularly reviewed by managers, governors and elected members concerned to establish open institutions. Other important factors in maintaining an open, safe culture are:

- the involvement of children, parents and staff in the governance of institutions, even residential homes;
- screening of staff against hard and 'soft' information systems;
- governors and elected members visiting and actively enquiring into the conduct of management and control;

- the presence of suitably screened outsiders as independent visitors and providers of leisure and creative activity;
- regular visits by social workers, professionals and specialists;
- private telephone facilities and access to helplines and help, with information on sources of help freely available;
- access to parents and relatives by phone as well as visits;
- good structures of pastoral care that involve children themselves;
- good staffing ratios at times when children and young people require support and supervision – after school, weekends, nights and mornings;
- regular inspections involving interviews with students, residents and parents to monitor care, and as a disincentive to sex offenders;
- clear information to students, residents and those entering foster care from the head of the home or the school, or the social worker about the behaviour they may expect from staff and carers.

If regimes of abuse can exist, then so too can regimes of decency, where care is taken to deal with young people's emotional well-being and they are offered respect. If children themselves are more involved in debate and discussion about their behaviour towards each other, serious lapses of trust by teachers, carers and fellow residents are more likely to come to light, acting as an impediment to sex offenders. Abusers admit that the possibility of getting caught is the greatest disincentive (Conte 1990; Dobash *et al.* 1993; Colton and Vanstone 1996).

Even with all this in place, we are unlikely to be able entirely to eliminate assaults. But there is no excuse for tolerating systems that give abusers easy access. Too many of the children reported here felt unloved and unwanted, were abused and could get no help. We simply must offer safer care to children as hurt and rejected as these.

References

Barter, C., Keep, G. and MacLeod, M. (1996) *Children at Crisis Point*, London: ChildLine.

Bridge Child Care Consultancy Service (1996) *In Care Contacts: The West Case: The Report of a Review of over 2,000 Files of Young Persons in Residential Care*, London: The Bridge Consultancy.

Colton, M. and Vanstone, M. (1996) *Betrayal of Trust: Sexual Abuse by Men who Work with Children*, London: Free Association Books.

Conte, J.R. (1990) 'The incest offender: An overview and introduction', in A.L. Horton, B.L. Johnson, L.M. Roundy and D. Williams (eds) *The Incest*

Perpetrator: The Family Member No-one Wants to Treat, Newbury Park: Sage.

Cowie, H. (1995) 'Approaches to peer support: Befriending, counselling and mediation', *Young Minds Newsletter* 23: 14–15.

Dartington Social Research Unit (1995) *Child Protection: Messages from Research*, London: HMSO.

Department of Education (1994) *Bullying – Don't Suffer in Silence. An Anti-bullying Pack for Schools*, London: HMSO.

Department for Education and Employment (1995) *Protecting Children from Abuse: The Role of the Education Service*, Circular number 10/95, London: HMSO.

Dobash, R.P., Carnie, J. and Waterhouse, L. (1993) 'Child sexual abusers: Recognition and response', in L. Waterhouse (ed.) *Child Abuse and Child Abusers*, London: Jessica Kingsley.

Epstein, C. (1995) *Listening to Ten-Year-Olds*, London: ChildLine.

—— (1996) 'You can do therapy on the telephone', *Young Minds* 29: 12–15.

Home Office, Department of Health, Department of Education and Science, Welsh Office (1991) *Working Together under the Children Act 1989: A Guide to Arrangements for Inter-Agency Co-operation for the Protection of Children from Abuse*, London: HMSO.

Keep, G. (1996) *Going to Court: Child Witnesses in their Own Words*, London: ChildLine.

Kelly, L., Burton, L. and Regan, S.I. (1991) 'An exploratory study of the prevalence of sexual abuse in a sample of 16–21 year olds', London: University of North London.

La Fontaine, J. and Morris, S. (1991) *The Boarding School Line*, London: ChildLine.

Lees, B., Morris, S. and Wheatley, H. (1994) *Time to Listen*, London: Child-Line.

Levy, A.C. and Kahan, B. (1991) *The Pindown Experience and the Protection of Children*, Staffordshire County Council.

MacLeod, M. (1996a) *Talking with Children about Child Abuse*, London: ChildLine.

—— (1996b) *Children and Racism*, London: ChildLine.

—— (1997) *Children Living Away From Home*, London: ChildLine.

MacLeod, M. and Barter, C. (1996) *We Know It's Tough to Talk*, London: ChildLine.

MacLeod, M. and Morris, S. (1996) *Why Me?*, London: ChildLine.

NSPCC (1996) *Childhood Matters: Report of the National Commission of Inquiry into the Prevention of Child Abuse*, London: The Stationery Office.

Sharp, S. and Smith, P.K. (1994) *Tackling Bullying in Your School: A Practical Handbook for Teachers*, London: Routledge.

Shaw, C. (1998) *Remember My Messages*, London: The Who Cares? Trust.

Smith, M., Bee, P., Heverin, A. and Nobes, G. (1995) *Parental Control Within the Family: The Nature and Extent of Parental Violence Towards Children*, London: Thomas Coram Foundation.

Smith, P.K. and Sharp, S. (1994) *School Bullying*, London: Routledge.

Suderman, M., Jaffe, P.G. and Hastings, E. (1993) *A.S.A.P.: A School-based Antiviolence Programme*, London, Ontario: London Family Court Clinic.

Tattum, D.P. and Herbert, G. (1993) *Countering Bullying*, Stoke-on-Trent: Trentham Books.

Utting, W. (1991) *Children in the Public Care: A Review of Residential Child Care*, London: HMSO.

—— (1997) *People Like Us: The Report of the Review of the Safeguards for Children Living Away from Home*, London: HMSO.

Warner, N. (1992) *Choosing with Care: The Report of the Committee of Enquiry into the Selection, Development and Management of Staff in Children's Homes*, London: HMSO.

3 Independent investigations into institutional child abuse

Developing theory and practice

Christine Barter

This chapter is based primarily upon recent research findings relating to child protection investigations into allegations of institutional abuse undertaken by the National Society for the Prevention of Cruelty to Children (NSPCC). Initially, it explores the lack of UK empirical evidence relating to institutional child abuse and the subsequent dependence on inquiry reports. Some implications of this reliance in relation to how institutional abuse has been both conceptualised and responded to are addressed. The North American experience and research evidence are drawn upon to illustrate the primary differences between investigating institutional abuse allegations and suspected familial abuse. Findings from the current research concerning the nature and dynamics of the institutional abuse allegations investigated are introduced. Following this, four main areas, perceived by investigators as having the most impact on the investigatory process, are explored. Finally, a number of procedural considerations derived from the research are presented.

Official guidance

The official guidance governing the investigation of out-of-home abuse in England and Wales is, at the time of writing, mainly contained in *Working Together under the Children Act 1989: A Guide to Arrangements for Inter-Agency Co-operation for the Protection of Children from Abuse* (Home Office *et al.* 1991). In this, the NSPCC is identified as being able to provide an increased element of independence to local authority investigations. It is this experience that the study explores.

At the time of writing this guidance is under Government review. The consultation paper highlights a number of factors in relation to out-of-home investigations. A major proposition for comment is the development of dedicated local groups of suitably trained and experienced police officers and social workers to undertake such investigations. The consultation paper also sets out a number of recommendations for consideration on procedures for vetting and selection of staff, and better avenues for complaint.

The current guidance, alongside an array of inquiries and reviews concerning institutional child abuse, asserts the significance of 'independence' within these investigations. The authoritative review by Sir William Utting on safeguards for children living away from home reinforces this importance, stating that:

> Investigations into allegations of abuse in foster care or residential settings differ significantly from investigations into allegations against parents or others in the child's own home. Social workers find themselves examining the actions of people regarded as co-workers or professional colleagues. If they are members of the same department, its management may wittingly or unwittingly obstruct the investigation because it is reluctant to have failures or weaknesses exposed or is unable to acknowledge the possibility of harmful misconduct by its employees.
>
> (1997: 182–3)

No further comment is provided on how independence should be operationally defined, established or maintained. Indeed, little substantial analysis of what this term actually means in practice has been undertaken. The above quotation also states that investigations into institutional compared to familial abuse are significantly different. However, once again, little examination has been undertaken to understand and respond to these differences.

The current research on which this chapter is based enabled a more detailed picture to emerge surrounding the investigation of institutional abuse allegations. The strength of this study resides in the wide range of investigations covered, from a single isolated event through to allegations of widespread sexual abuse. This is in contrast to previous texts, for example Brannan *et al.* (1993), which specifically focus on large-scale abuse investigations. While we should obviously be cautious in making generalisations from a single agency's experience, distinct lessons can be drawn from it that are relevant to child protection practice generally.

The wider context of institutional abuse

Although there has been significant public and professional concern surrounding the abuse of children in out-of-home settings, this focus has not been mirrored in research. Consequently, in this country, few studies have critically explored the nature and dynamics of institutional abuse of children in its wider context. Some small exploratory studies have emerged (for example Westcott and Clément 1992; Safe and Sound 1995; Colton and Vanstone 1996) and some wider studies surrounding out-of-home settings have incorporated aspects of child protection (Berridge and Brodie 1998; Sinclair and Gibbs 1998). Due to this dearth of empirical evidence our understanding of this form of child abuse has predominantly been shaped by inquiry reports, as Stanley notes in Chapter 1, which have appeared with depressing regularity over the last decade. These have predominantly, although not exclusively, surrounded the organised sexual and physical abuse of children, frequently boys, by male workers and managers.

Such inquiries are characterised by the extent of abuse investigated. Indeed, it is the atrocious magnitude of abuse that shocks both the public and professionals alike. The strength of these inquiries lies in their detail and analysis of immediate events, including contexts leading to abuse and in their practical recommendations (Stein 1993). Collectively, these inquiry reports represent an impressive body of information. For example, Berridge and Brodie (1996) concentrating on three inquiry reports, identify a range of common management, policy and practice factors associated with the abuse.

Nevertheless, inquiry reports exhibit severe limitations in relation to understanding more widely the concept of child abuse and neglect in residential settings. The most predominant being that, by their very nature, they focus solely upon examining widespread, generally organised, abuse. In addition, the domination of sexual abuse has meant that other forms of institutional abuse and neglect have rarely received the same level of analysis or comment, even though research in North America has clearly demonstrated that sexual abuse is not the most common form of institutional maltreatment suffered by children (Groze 1990; Rosenthal *et al.* 1991; Blatt 1992). Similarly, Utting (1997) states that, although the dangers of paedophiles should not be understated, we must not become so preoccupied that the other hazards children encounter in out-of-home care are discounted or neglected.

Consequently, we must question how representative of the general dynamics of institutional abuse these 'extreme' cases are. Obviously, the lessons learnt must inform policy and practice, although the degree to which previous recommendations have been acted upon is debatable (Stein 1993). However, unless we also develop a more multifaceted conceptualisation and understanding of the nature of institutional abuse the effectiveness of different protective procedures and mechanisms, including independent investigations, will remain unclear.

Furthermore, it is important to recognise that current understandings of institutional abuse and neglect have been characterised by a model of 'individual pathological blame' (Jones and Myers 1997). Thus, when abuse has been exposed it is not viewed as a problem of society, or even organisations, but of individuals. This has implications for both recognising and responding to abuse incidents in out-of-home settings. It is imperative that the initial response to an allegation of institutional abuse is to believe that the incident could have happened (Barter 1998). However, the individualisation of institutional abuse means that establishments that have introduced prevention measures can come to perceive themselves as being immune from the dangers of abuse, and consequently dismiss allegations when they arise. In North America, Bloom (1992) identifies a commonly held belief that only 'bad agencies', employing 'sick' people were involved in institutional abuse allegations. In reality, even if exceptional risk management policies and practices have been implemented, this will not free the agency from the possibility of abuse.

The emphasis on pathological individuals has also suppressed the development of a more critical conceptualisation that positions institutional child abuse within wider structures of inequality, including gender, ethnicity, disability and ultimately generational inequalities between children and adults. As Frost and Stein (1989) assert, it is difficult to make sense of the experiences of children and young people without recognising the construction of childhood as a period of dependency and powerlessness.

This individualisation of blame has resulted in preventive strategies focusing on reducing the risk of abuse, through for example better screening and training of staff, rather than focusing on strategies to empower children (Cawson 1997). Indeed, as Stanley points out in Chapter 1, children's rights perspectives have often been met with varying degrees of scepticism and hostility (Barter 1997; Utting 1997).

Due to this lack of theoretical and empirical interest in the institutional abuse of children, many of the research and social work texts that underpin the present study originate from North America, where many states have developed specialised teams to investigate this form of abuse. However, we need to be cautious when transferring findings based on the American experience. The nature of US institutions are substantially different to our own, as are the wider social and cultural forces in which institutions are embedded. These factors need to be taken into account when viewing the North American research evidence presented in the following section of this chapter.

Differences between investigating institutional and familial abuse allegations

Research from the US consistently highlights the differences between intra-familial and institutional abuse investigations, and the problems associated with 'stretching' familial investigation procedures and techniques to fit institutional settings (Nunno 1997). Within the literature a range of factors have been identified that are unique to the investigation of institutional abuse and neglect allegations, and these are presented below. However, before looking in depth at these factors, it is important to recognise that significant similarities do exist between these two forms of investigation (Durkin 1982). Westcott (1991) surmises that aspects shared by both include isolation, unequal power relationships and denial of abuse. Child protection professionals are therefore not confronting an entirely unknown phenomenon when investigating abuse in out-of-home settings. Five main differences are explored below.

The nature and dynamics of institutional abuse

The most obvious departure from familial abuse relates to the nature and dynamics of the abuse itself. Many factors distinguish the nature of out-of-home abuse from other forms of maltreatment, the most fundamental being the setting itself, where care and treatment are provided within a formally organised environment (Westcott 1991), in which unrelated adults and children are placed together.

Westcott (1993), while acknowledging that residential care can be a positive experience for children, also identifies that institutional care can itself be a risk factor for abuse. The dynamics of institutional settings can lead to a climate in which children are particularly vulnerable to being abused. Lerman (1994), on reviewing the available data, concludes that children in out-of-home placements have a greater or equal chance of being victimised by maltreatment than children living in their family homes. Furthermore, children in residential care are not open to the same degree of external scrutiny through relatives, family friends and neighbours as are children in families. Thus, not only are children in institutional settings more vulnerable to maltreatment than those living in families, but opportunities for the abuse to be externally observed and reported are also diminished.

Standard of care

Staff working with children are held to a higher standard of care than parents (Rosenthal *et al.* 1991); parents have a heightened level of discretion in their child-rearing practices compared to residential workers, including the level of basic care, supervision and methods of control. In addition, the severity of the abuse incident in out-of-home care is irrelevant to whether an investigation is needed, as the organisational context should safeguard and protect children's welfare at all times (Thomas 1990).

Wilful intent

Out-of-home maltreatment also differs from familial abuse in relation to the issue of wilful intent. The State Institutional Abuse and Neglect Advisory Committee (1987) in Colorado, USA, found that mitigating circumstances and intent are not relevant criteria for determining child abuse and/or neglect in residential settings. Facilities must ensure in advance that the childcare environment is harm free – it is therefore immaterial if the abuse occurred accidentally or that mitigating circumstances were present.

Culpability

A further distinction lies in the scope of culpability. This is significantly greater in out-of-home child protection investigations, extending from identifying the 'direct' abuser or abusers to including those responsible for managing the facility. The investigators also need to determine if the problem is administratively re-addressable (Nunno and Motz 1988), for example through the introduction of new or enhanced policies or procedures to safeguard children and young people against similar abuse scenarios.

Role of institutional investigations

The accumulation of the above factors means that major distinctions exist in both the role and function of institutional compared to familial investigations. Kelleher (1987) describes an agency's response

to familial abuse as following models of responding both to the immediate abuse incident and to supporting the family unit after the
incident has been substantiated. Although these response models may
be imperfect, they attempt to deal not only with the abuse incident but
with the reintegration of the child into the family unit by assisting the
family to prevent further abuse situations occurring. In contrast, the
aim of independent investigations is to decide if it is probable that the
abuse did or did not occur, and to identify the person or persons
responsible. The goal is not the development of a treatment
programme nor the establishment of an effective identification with
either party (Bloom 1992). Although prevention may be an aspect, it is
not the primary or overriding purpose of the investigation, and this is
reflected in the investigation process (Kelleher 1987).

Current research findings

Methodology

The research to be described here (Barter 1998) entailed interviewing
all NSPCC practitioners who had undertaken an investigation
concerning abuse in a residential or day care setting between 1994 and
1996. Due to the time constraints of the project, it was not possible to
include the views and evaluations of either the young people involved
in the investigations, or the commissioning local authorities. Both
would have provided valuable insights. A total of forty-one semi-struc-
tured interviews were conducted, and thirty-six investigation reports
undertaken over the two-year period were also analysed, the main
findings of which are presented below. These reports obviously
comprise a non-representative sample, and their findings are not necessarily indicative of the national picture regarding either incidence or
the nature of institutional abuse. Previous research findings, mainly
derived from the American experience, are provided for comparison.

Characteristics of the investigations

The thirty-six investigation reports involved sixty-seven children,
making a total of seventy-six allegations, against forty members of
staff and ten other residents, within thirty-seven settings (the majority
being residential children's homes).

Twenty-four of the investigations concerned allegations about
present abuse, eight related to past abuse, and four to both past and
present abuse. The length of investigations, from initial strategy

meeting to completion of the investigation ranged between three days to ten months, with the modal length of time being between three to four weeks. The highest number of children involved in any one investigation was fifteen; however, the great majority (twenty-five) involved only a single child.

Just over half (forty-one) of the children's allegations were upheld by the investigation team. However, in nearly a third (twenty-seven) the outcome of the investigation was inconclusive, with nine deemed to be untrue. The low level of substantiation of institutional abuse allegations has been a cause of concern within the US (Groze 1990; Nunno and Rindfleisch 1991). In comparison, the level of 54 per cent found within the present study appears to be relatively high. As the current research focused upon the process of the investigation itself rather than the actual abuse incidents, all reports were analysed irrespective of their outcomes.

Characteristics of the children

Of the sixty-seven children involved in the investigations, thirty-four were boys and thirty-three were girls. Over half of the children were aged between 14 and 15 years, with over two-thirds being between the ages of 13 and 16. Similarly, US research has overwhelmingly found that the vast majority of children experiencing out-of-home abuse are adolescents (Groze 1990), which reflects the general ages of the resident population surveyed (Blatt 1992).

Characteristics of the alleged abusers

Table 3.1 clearly shows that more male than female staff were implicated in the abuse allegations. If this is viewed alongside the fact that the majority of residential work is undertaken by a female workforce (Balloch *et al.* 1995; Berridge and Brodie 1998) it is clear that males are proportionally over-represented. Table 3.1 also illustrates that the majority of allegations were against workers of direct-care level, although managers were also subject to accusations, albeit less frequently.

Previous research has confirmed that males are proportionally over-represented as perpetrators of institutional abuse (Rindfleisch and Baros-Van Hull 1982; Blatt 1992), and that the majority of reported abusers are direct-care workers (Sundrum 1984; Blatt 1990). Earlier studies have provided an array of key variables or risk factors associated with institutional abuse, many relating specifically to staff at

Table 3.1 Position of alleged abuser by gender

Position of alleged abuser	Male	Female	Total
Residential direct-care workers	21	9	30
Residents	9	1	10
Officer in charge	5	0	5
Assistant officer in charge	2	0	2
Domestic staff	0	2	2
External persons	1	0	1
Total	38	12	50

direct care level (Nunno 1997). In addition, a small number of investigations (three) concerned abuse by other residents. However, past research has indicated that abuse by residents may be more pronounced than is reflected in this study (Lunn 1990; Westcott and Clément 1992). Possible explanations for the low level of investigations concerning children as abusers have been explored elsewhere (see Barter 1997).

Type of abuse allegations

Table 3.2 shows that the most frequently investigated allegations concerned physical abuse, followed by sexual abuse. Together, these constitute two-thirds of all allegation types. The use of inappropriate restraint was alleged by nearly a quarter of children in this sample. Differential patterns of abuse allegations were found to exist for male and female children. Most of the allegations made by boys concerned physical abuse, while allegations by girls more often concerned sexual abuse.

Within the US research, no clear pattern has emerged regarding the type of abuse children in residential facilities most commonly experience (see Blatt 1992; Groze 1990; Rosenthal *et al.* 1991). However, the relationship found within the present study between a child's gender and the type of out-of-home abuse experienced has been widely identified in the literature (Groze 1990; Rosenthal *et al.* 1991). Interestingly, this is in contrast to many of the inquiries in the UK that have focused on the sexual abuse of boys (see Kirkwood 1993; Barratt 1998).

Table 3.2 Type of institutional abuse allegation by gender of child

Abuse type	Male	Female	Total
Physical abuse only	20	6	26
Sexual abuse only	4	13	17
Restraint only	8	4	12
Physical and sexual abuse*	0	5	5
Physical abuse and restraint*	1	1	2
Sexual abuse and restraint*	0	2	2
Neglect/inappropriate care	1	2	3
Total	34	33	67

Note: *represents more than one type of allegation by individual children

Interview findings

Although the interview data covered a wide range of issues, the subsequent discussion will focus primarily on four central areas identified by investigators as being key to undertaking sensitive and appropriate investigations.

Remit and scope

The remit and scope of the investigation was a central concern of many respondents, and mostly this focused on how encompassing the scope of the investigation should be. The majority of respondents (twenty-six) who expressed a view felt that the remit should not simply focus on the specific incident but needed to be more extensive, thus enabling the wider dynamics of the establishment, including the role of management, to be evaluated within the child protection investigation.

A minority (nine) felt that it should be 'brief focused', as they were investigating a specific incident by an individual member of staff. This very narrow approach may not allow the multifactorial causes that frequently underlie institutional abuse to be uncovered. In the worst-case scenario this stance may miss the widespread abuse of children within an institution. The current research found that in five cases widespread abuse was discovered when the original complaint involved only an individual child and abuser.

Kelleher (1987) has criticised this single incident approach as 'crisis management' and argues that the focus should be on improving the total system, as opposed to examining a particular allegation. Similarly, Grayson (1988) has emphasised an ecological approach that can move investigations beyond probing a particular incident to examining the quality of life for all residents.

This research found that in practice many respondents (twenty-four) considered that the investigations' remits had sometimes been too restrictive, especially in relation to including management in the investigations. In other instances, investigators had no authority to interview routinely all members of staff or children in the facility. The problems surrounding 'whistle-blowing' may still be very pertinent if staff have evidence about an allegation but fear possible reprisals if they are seen to approach an investigation team. By automatically interviewing all staff this reduces the need for staff to take the initiative individually.

In a number of cases, workers who initially seemed to have no direct knowledge about an incident were able to provide important information when interviewed. Each investigation's remit must therefore be decided on its own merits, without any external pressure or restrictions.

Independence

This current research also indicates that the concept of independence should not be viewed in a simplistic manner. Even though NSPCC investigators are not directly employed by the commissioning local authorities, over three-quarters still viewed their level of independence as being of some concern. It is important to place these anxieties in context before looking at them in detail. All investigators felt they were able to bring greater levels of independence compared to commissioning local authorities' own child protection workers. Respondents also stressed that the children who had made allegations about abuse generally felt that the involvement of the NSPCC meant that they were being taken seriously by the authority concerned. Additionally, many young people had spontaneously told investigators that they were pleased the NSPCC were involved, as they were not directly connected with the facility and consequently would not be biased.

Nevertheless, half of respondents reported feeling worried that they might jeopardise their projects' relationships with the local authority if they 'rocked the boat too much' within the investigation. This was of particular concern to projects that had established service-level agreements. This is echoed by Francis who warns that more and more voluntary organisations are expressing their dissatisfaction with the contract culture, stressing that:

The quest by local authorities to get the best deal from contracts with the voluntary sector seems to be eroding the fundamental principle of partnership. The casualties will not only be voluntary sector creativity and independence, but the clients the services are meant to support.

(1996: 27)

In a small number of instances, respondents felt that local authorities had approached them with a firmly set agenda that restricted their ability to undertake a comprehensive investigation, but which they had felt pressurised to accept.

A related problem associated with the investigator's ability to undertake an 'independent' investigation concerned investigating other professionals. The most commonly stated problem concerned investigating professionals within the team's own geographical area. This was additionally compounded in many cases by investigating professionals who were working in a field related to their own. Respondents were particularly uncomfortable with investigating professionals whom they knew through their general work.

Nearly a third of respondents (thirteen) felt that having previous contact with a residential establishment, even if this did not include direct contact with the alleged abuser(s), might affect their ability to view the situation objectively. Primarily, this concern centred upon bringing prior knowledge and preconceptions about a facility into the investigation, which might affect their impartiality. This highlights the importance of ensuring that preliminary discussions are thorough enough for independent agencies to be clear about the level of commitment needed, and that no possible conflict of interest is present. Present protocols already in place to ensure the independence of such investigations need to be built upon. These should include procedures not only to involve an external agency but also to ensure they are the most appropriate. The research indicated that agencies should not be involved in this role if:

- the team has significant service-level contracts with the commissioning authority in relation to other services;
- the project has ongoing contact with the establishment concerned or may have contact in the future;
- the team has no knowledge of residential-care procedures and practices;
- the team has no experience of undertaking investigations into allegations of child abuse;

- the project can only release workers for very limited periods of time due to other planned work commitments.

Support

The provision of support in an investigation was universally viewed as paramount in ensuring its smooth running and in reducing the stress and anxiety experienced by all those involved. However, three-quarters of respondents judged the provision of support provided to be inadequate.

Supporting the alleged victim

Three-quarters of respondents talked about their anxiety surrounding the lack of support for the child or children involved. Often, this placed investigators in the difficult position of having to support the child whilst undertaking the investigation, placing their neutrality in jeopardy. This also meant that, due to the pressures involved in these forms of investigations, the level of commitment needed by that young person could not be met by the investigators. This often left the young person feeling isolated, confused, angry and not listened to.

Investigators stated that this support should include one-to-one counselling (although the impact on the child's ability to be a credible witness in criminal proceedings must be acknowledged), provision of information about the investigation process, updating the young person regarding the investigation, and consulting with the young person to ascertain his or her views and wishes. Support should be provided from the very beginning to ensure that children feel confident about making the complaint, and reduce the risk of them withdrawing their allegation due to pressure or uncertainty about the investigation procedures (Safe and Sound 1995). Additionally, it should continue even when the investigation has been completed, irrespective of outcome, until it is no longer required by the child.

The research found general agreement that children's advocacy officers were the most appropriate providers of this support. The strengths of this service, as the Leicestershire Inquiry (Kirkwood 1993) found, lie in its ability to be semi-independent, situated outside the formal line management structure and being directly accountable only to the deputy director, thus bypassing other levels of the hierarchy.

Supporting the alleged abuser

The research showed that only rarely did the local authority appoint a formal link person for the alleged abuser. Even in instances where the local authority did provide such support this was often limited. Frequently, the support seemed to recede as the investigation proceeded. The absence of this provision in many of the cases examined meant that investigation teams were providing advice and support not simply to the child, but also to the alleged abuser – an obviously unacceptable position. Respondents felt that the resulting isolation significantly added to the pressure these workers were already experiencing, and in some instances created heightened hostility, consequently making the investigation more difficult.

Inquiry reports have previously identified the enormous stress that workers are under while they are being investigated. The Oxendon House inquiry report (Roycroft 1994) stated that following the closure of the home in question, almost all of the staff suffered ill health and in a number of cases 'acute stress' was reported. It is the responsibility of senior line managers to ensure that the worker's interests are protected, to organise representation via the trade union or staff association, update the person on the investigation's progress and secure professional counselling if required.

Supporting other children

Respondents also felt that other young people within the settings were not being properly supported through the process. Allegations of abuse may be particularly difficult for vulnerable children to deal with, especially if they raise issues relating to the children's own past abuse. Obviously, the primary source of support for the young people is through the establishment's staff group.

Supporting the staff group

Respondents often felt that staff reacted with incredulity about the allegation, perceiving it as an over-reaction. A number of investigators reported experiencing a lack of co-operation and hostility, with some residential staff being unhelpful, manipulative and derisory. Respondents reported various tactics. For example, some respondents felt that the staff had deliberately 'wound children up' directly before they were due to interview them, making them unmanageable in the meeting.

However, investigators also reported that facilities were often simply 'left to get on with it', being offered very little, if any, support from their immediate line managers. Nor was advice or guidance routinely offered regarding their responsibility for supporting the alleged victim and the wider resident group of children. This is important, as the staff group may experience great difficulties believing the child, and consequently workers may try to dissuade the child from holding to their allegation, or distance themselves emotionally (Bloom 1992).

This research suggests that open communication is an essential element in an effective investigation, as it reduces anxiety and serves to mobilise the collaboration of the facility's wider staff group. Consequently, the staff team should be told clearly and unambiguously what has been done, including how the worker is being supported, and what will be done in response to the allegation. However, if the abuse is thought to be pervasive throughout a facility, open communication may be detrimental, alerting abusers to the need to devise alibis and disguise possible indicators of abuse.

Furthermore, respondents generally felt that priority should be given to emphasising that the staff's main responsibility is to safeguard the welfare of, and provide support to, the alleged victim. A certain amount of staff members' anxiety may be related to their concern about how the children will react to them and what is the most appropriate response. Investigators felt that in-service training on responding to abuse allegations would be beneficial for many residential workers and may serve to focus supportive attention on the complainant as well as the wider resident group.

Supporting and working with the family

The child's family should be informed of the child's allegations and what is being done, including a description of how the child is being protected and helped through the crisis, and what services are being provided (Bloom 1992). The family must be helped to support the child, even if they do not believe the allegation is true. The family may also have to deal with past incidents of abuse that may re-emerge due to the present allegations. This may need specialist expertise.

Post-substantiation issues

Most respondents (thirty-one) felt that a central feature of an investigation was to identify which policies, procedures and working practices may have contributed to the abuse occurring. Leading on from this, over half of respondents felt that the final report should not simply identify the present policy and practice issues, but ought to contain specific recommendations as to how these could be changed, to ensure that the abuse would not reoccur for similar reasons.

However, many respondents (thirty-three) found that the post-substantiation phase of the investigation was 'unsatisfactory', 'highly frustrating' or 'inadequate'. Most felt that, in comparison to investigating intra-familial abuse, there existed a lack of post-substantiation procedures.

In many cases a formalised process to present the findings of the report, including any recommendations and to evaluate the investigation process itself, was agreed at the initial strategy meeting. However, in eight cases, local authority representatives had either failed to attend these meetings or their representative was not of adequate seniority to comment on the recommendations.

In some instances (eleven) the local authority concerned had welcomed the report's recommendations concerning practice and policy initiatives. It was felt that these local authorities viewed their recommendations as positive contributions to their procedures relating to protecting children from abuse within their residential facilities. However, most of these respondents were unsure as to what extent local authorities had considered their practices and policies in response to the recommendations.

Generally, once the local authority received the investigation report, little or no further contact occurred meaning that most of those interviewed were unable to say if any changes to policy or practice had followed their recommendations. However, as most respondents believed that the local authority had not been especially receptive to the reports' recommendations, it was thought unlikely that they would be implemented. One project, for example, had undertaken two separate investigations into the same residential establishment. It was felt that the local authority concerned had not implemented many of the recommendations contained in the initial investigation report, as similar problems relating to practice and procedures were still present in the institution when a second investigation was undertaken.

The fact that the study has highlighted the inadequate procedures for presenting recommendations and the apparent lack of commitment shown by some of the local authorities concerned, raises serious concerns about how adequately some children are being protected.

This experience is reflected in the US literature. Grayson (1988) found that US practitioners evaluated the intervention phase of these investigations as being frustrating and limited. Kelleher (1987) also highlights the problem of intervention. With intra-familial abuse, agencies follow models of responding both to the immediate abuse incident and to supporting the family unit after the incident had been substantiated. Although these response models may be imperfect, she argues that at least they attempt not only to deal with the incident but also with the development of strategies to prevent the abuse reoccurring, and the reintegration of the child into the family unit. The same author reports that when abuse occurs in an institution response models are more limited. In these cases the response is directed towards determining if the abuse incident occurred, with little attention beyond the investigation and substantiation of the incident. Thus, whilst there is a post-substantiation model for family abuse, no complementary model exists for institutional abuse. Bloom (1992) stresses that the abusive situation should serve as a signal to initiate a risk management analysis of the agency, although he notes that this is rarely done.

The current research suggests that an additional external element may be necessary to guarantee that local authorities fulfil their post-substantiation role. One possible solution may be for all reports to be presented to the Area Child Protection Committee, which would then be in a position to evaluate the recommendations and monitor their implementation. Another option may be to involve the Social Services Inspectorate, which could provide an overview in a similar manner.

Conclusion

This chapter has highlighted the lack of empirical evidence relating to the institutional abuse of children. This has not only stifled theoretical understanding but has impeded the development of both policy and practice initiatives. The problems surrounding the subsequent reliance on inquiry reports have been briefly explored, including the dangers of exclusively reproducing models of individual pathological blame. Some of the main research findings derived from a recent study of investigations into institutional abuse allegations have been presented. The major problems associated with these forms of investigations have been documented and some possible solutions offered. Obviously, the limitations of the research mean that the emergent messages for policy and practice are tentative. Nevertheless, it is hoped that the research will raise the need for a more informed and critical debate to emerge regarding the nature and role of these investigations. The necessity to ensure that independence is both theoretically and operationally defined and maintained, has been emphasised, as has the need to guarantee that all those involved in these investigations, whether directly or indirectly, receive the support they require. The importance of ensuring that the post-substantiation stage of these investigations is not viewed by the commissioning authority as an optional extra, but as an intrinsic aspect of the investigatory process, has been clearly reported. Ultimately, until a mandatory national mechanism exists to monitor and report on these types of investigations, our understanding and consequently our responses will be sadly lacking. Finally, a number of procedural considerations relating to good practice were identified in the research, and these are summarised below.

Procedural considerations

Policy developments

An operational definition of institutional abuse and neglect must be agreed.

Criteria for 'independence' determined and appropriate agencies identified.

Joint training for police, social workers and independent investigators developed and implemented.

Procedures distributed to residential workers, young people and their parents.

Evaluation and formal follow-up procedures regarding recommendations should be developed and implemented.

The post-substantiation stage of the process must be clearly defined as central to the investigation process.

Immediate action in response to an allegation

Ensure that the complainant is safe, and that no other children or young people are in need of protection.

Consideration should be given to suspending the worker, or moving them to a non-contact role.

Indications of administration or management involvement in the alleged incident(s) should be explored at this stage.

The child's family should be informed of the allegation.

Strategy meeting

In line with official guidance a strategy meeting should be convened, no later than the following day, to plan and co-ordinate the investigation. The group should meet periodically throughout the investigation to evaluate progress and discuss any difficulties. Representatives should be of senior status, with at least a deputy or assistant director of social services attending. This group should have the authority to allocate resources as necessary.

Remit

The scope of an investigation should be ultimately determined by the investigators to ensure that independence is maintained throughout the investigation.

A key senior local-authority representative should be identified and informed of changes to an investigation's scope and subsequent resource requirements.

Any significant changes to an investigation's scope, especially the involvement of other workers in the abuse, or other settings should trigger a strategy meeting to ensure that present protection plans are adequate.

Resources

The provision of adequate administrative back-up is essential, especially if past residents need to be traced and contacted.

The team should include a gender and ethnicity balance so that young people can have a genuine choice of who interviews them.

Support requirements should be evaluated and allocated for all those involved in the investigation process.

Evidence collecting

Interviews should be undertaken in accordance with the Home Office's (1991) *Memorandum of Good Practice*.

All interviews should be recorded and transcribed 'verbatim'.

Statements should be read by, or to, the witness, who should be asked to sign the statement as a true representation of their account.

Post-investigation meeting

This should be viewed as a central aspect of the investigation process, and all the strategy team should attend.

The final report presented at this meeting should state if the allegation has been found to be:

- substantiated;
- inconclusive 'but with concern' (where the allegation has not been substantiated but where child protection concerns relating to the workers' general working practices emerged);
- inconclusive;
- false.

Substantiated and inconclusive 'but with concern' outcomes should be accompanied with a detailed breakdown of the following issues:

- assessment of culpability of wider staff group and management;
- identification of any policies, procedures, safeguards and working practices that either directly or indirectly facilitated or enabled the abuse to occur;
- recommendations regarding how policies, procedures and practices should be modified or changed to ensure that abuse does not occur in the future.

This meeting should also evaluate the investigation process itself to determine if procedures need to be revised or changed. Young people's evaluations should be sought so that they can inform good practice.

The young person should be told personally of the outcome by the investigators and receive a formal letter from the director, deputy or assistant director of social services.

Acknowledgement

The author would like to thank Professor David Berridge for his comments on an earlier draft of this chapter.

References

Balloch, S., Andrew, T., Ginn, J., McLean, J., Pahl, J. and Williams, J. (1995) *Working in the Social Services*, London: National Institute for Social Work, Research Unit.

Barratt, J. (1998) *Report into 'the Trotter affair': Report by J.K. Barratt to the Council of the London Borough of Hackney*, London: Council of the London Borough of Hackney.

Barter, C. (1997) 'Who's to blame: Conceptualising institutional abuse by children', *Early Child Development and Care* 133: 101–14.

—— (1998) *Investigating Institutional Abuse of Children: An Exploration of the NSPCC Experience*, London: NSPCC.

Berridge, D. and Brodie, I. (1996) 'Residential child care in England and Wales: The inquiries and after', in M. Hill and J. Aldgate (eds) *Child Welfare Services: Developments in Law, Policy, Practice and Research*, London: Jessica Kingsley.

—— (1998) *Children's Homes Revisited*, London: Jessica Kingsley.

Blatt, E. (1990) 'Staff supervision and the prevention of institutional abuse and neglect in residential care settings', *Journal of Child and Youth Care* 4: 73–80.

—— (1992) 'Factors associated with child abuse and neglect in residential care settings', *Children and Youth Services Review* 14: 493–517.

Bloom, R.B. (1992) 'When staff members sexually abuse children in residential care', *Child Welfare League of America* LXXI(2): 131–45. Article based on paper presented at the annual meeting of the American Association of Children's Residential Centres in St. Petersburg, FL, November 1990.

Brannan, C., Jones, J.R. and Murch, J.D. (1993) *Castle Hill Report: Practice Guide*, Shrewsbury: Shropshire County Council.

Cawson, P. (1997) 'Who will guard the guards? Some questions about the models of inspection for residential settings with relevance to the protection of children from abuse by staff', *Early Child Development and Care* 133: 57–72.

Colton, M. and Vanstone, M. (1996) *Betrayal of Trust: Sexual Abuse by Men who Work with Children … In Their Own Words*, London: Free Association Books.

Durkin, R. (1982) 'Institutional child abuse from a family systems perspective: A working paper', in R. Hanson (ed.) *Institutional Abuse of Children and Youth*, New York: The Haworth Press.

Francis, J. (1996) 'Creative casualties', *Community Care*, 12–18 September: 26–7.

Frost, N. and Stein, M. (1989) *The Politics of Child Welfare: Inequalities, Power and Change*, London: Harvester Wheatsheaf.

Grayson, J. (1988) 'Abuse and neglect in out-of-home care', *Virginia Child Protection Newsletter* 25, Spring 1988, Virginia: Department of Social Services, Bureau of Child Protection Services.

Groze, V. (1990) 'An exploratory investigation into institutional mistreatment', *Children and Youth Services Review* 12: 229–41.

Home Office, Department of Health, Department of Education and Science, Welsh Office (1991) *Working Together under the Children Act 1989: A Guide to Arrangements for Inter-agency Co-operation for the Protection of Children from Abuse*, London: HMSO.

Home Office in conjunction with Department of Health (1992) *Memorandum of Good Practice on Video Recorded Interviews with Child Witnesses for Criminal Proceedings*, London: HMSO.

Jones, J. and Myers, J. (1997) 'The future detection and prevention of institutional abuse: Giving children a chance to participate in research', *Early Child Development and Care* 133: 115–25.

Kelleher, M.E. (1987) 'Investigating institutional abuse: A post-substantiation model', *Child Welfare* 4(6): 343–51.

Kirkwood, A. (1993) The Leicestershire Inquiry 1992, Leicester: Leicestershire County Council.

Lerman, P. (1994) 'Child protection and out-of-home care: System reforms and regulating placements', in G.B. Melton and F.D. Barry (eds) *Protecting Children from Abuse and Neglect: Foundations for National Strategy*, New York: Guildford Press.

Lunn, T. (1990) 'Pioneers of abuse control', *Social Work Today* 3(22): 9 (September 13).

Matsushima, J. (1990) 'Interviewing for alleged abuse in the residential treatment centre', *Child Welfare* 69: 321–31.

Mercer, M. (1982) 'Closing the barn door: the prevention of institutional abuse through standards', *Child and Youth Services* 4: 127–32.

Nunno, M. (1997) 'Institutional abuse: The role of leadership, authority and the environment in the social sciences literature', *Early Child Development and Care* 133: 21–40.

Nunno, M. and Motz, J. (1998) 'The development of an effective response to the abuse of children in out-of-home care', *Child Abuse and Neglect* 12: 521–8.

Nunno, M. and Rindfleisch, N. (1991) 'The abuse of children in out of home care', *Children and Society* 5(4): 295–305.

Rindfleisch, N. and Baros-Van Hull, J. (1982) 'Direct careworkers' attitudes toward the use of physical force with children', *Child and Youth Services* 4: 115–25.

Rosenthal, J., Motz, J., Edmonson, D. and Groze, V. (1991) 'A descriptive study of abuse and neglect in out of home placement', *Child Abuse and Neglect: The International Journal* 15: 249–60.

Roycroft, B. (1994) *Oxendon House: A Case to Answer? Report of the Independent Inquiry*, Bedfordshire County Council, August 1994.

Safe and Sound (1995) *So Who are We Meant to Trust Now?*, London: NSPCC.

Sinclair, I. and Gibbs, I. (1998) *Children's Homes: A Study in Diversity*, Chichester: Wiley.

State Institutional Abuse and Neglect Advisory Committee (1987) 'Specialized training in the investigation of out-of-home child abuse and neglect', Colorado: Department of Social Services, Division of Family and Children's Services. Paper prepared for the Interagency Project on Preventing Abuses in Out-of-Home Child Care Settings.

Stein, M (1993) 'The abuses and uses of residential child care', in H. Ferguson, R. Gilligan and R. Tordode (eds) *Surviving Childhood Adversity: Issues for Policy and Practice*, Dublin: Social Studies Press, Trinity College Dublin.

Sundrum, C. (1984) 'Obstacles to reducing patient abuse in public institutions', *Hospital and Community Psychiatry* 35: 238–43.

Thomas, G. (1990) 'Institutional child abuse, the making and prevention of an un-problem', *Journal of Child and Youth Care* 4(6): 1–22.

Utting, W. (1997) *People Like Us: The Report of The Review of the Safeguards for Children Living Away From Home*, London: HMSO.

Westcott, H. (1991) *Institutional Abuse of Children – From Research to Policy: A Review*, London: NSPCC.

—— (1993) *Abuse of Children and Adults with Disabilities*, London: NSPCC.

Westcott, H. and Clément, M. (1992) *NSPCC Experience of Child Abuse in Residential Care and Educational Placements: Results of a Survey*, London: NSPCC.

Williams, G. and McCreadie, J. (1992) *Ty Mawr Community Home Inquiry*, Cwmbran: Gwent County Council.

4 Abuse of people with learning disabilities

Layers of concern and analysis

Hilary Brown

This chapter provides an overview of abuse as an issue in the lives of people with learning disabilities, and of 'adult protection' as a role in, and for, service agencies. Although the focus is primarily on abuse in institutions, it is important to note that abuse also occurs at home and in the wider community. Abuse might be what triggers admission to more sheltered or institutional service provision (Barron 1996), as indeed might abusing behaviour on the part of service users living in community-based settings (Campbell *et al.* 1982; Jupp 1991). Williams (1993) has suggested that 'abuse' as a term minimises the impact of incidents that are often serious criminal offences, such as theft, assault or rape, while others have argued that the term sensationalises relatively minor occurrences, insults and injuries. It would seem that people with learning disabilities have always been at risk in services, in their families and in their wider communities, so it is important to maintain a critical stance towards the current heightened concern about their vulnerability and question why it has emerged in this way and at this time. The bottom line will be if increased awareness leads to useful interventions in service culture and organisation.

The discourse of 'abuse' is now being used to challenge a wide range of acts and practices, including violence and intimidation, non-consenting sexual acts, the bullying of less resilient people by more able service users, unacceptably deprived physical or social environments and financial exploitation or fraud. Some argue that it should include all abuses of human rights. Clearly, these issues are not new as the following chapter illustrates, and historically some of these practices have been hidden within service cultures while others have been quite open but variously rationalised as 'behaviour modification', 'relationships', 'control and restraint', or 'not giving in to attention seeking'. Abuse was regarded as a central, and inevitable, feature of institutionalised provision in influential models such as that of

Goffman (1961) and Wolfensberger (1975 and 1980) within an analysis whose focus was on organisations and ideology. The new discourse is much more personalised and within it the focus is on the experience of the *victim*.

This has some advantages for individuals and highlights some dilemmas for service organisations. It makes clear that people with learning disabilities are harmed, as any individual would be, by personal or sexual violence or exploitation. Harm is deemed equivalent whoever has caused it, for example whether it has been perpetrated by another service user, a member of staff or a stranger. This way of framing harmful acts highlights conflicts of interest *between* service users: the discourse of 'challenging behaviour' for example, designed to neutralise the stigma of difficult behaviour, inadvertently deflects from and discounts the experience of those on the receiving end of difficult behaviour. Naming these acts as abusive confronts service agencies with the need for specialised, safe (expensive) placements for those who present a risk to others. Men with learning disabilities who have difficult sexual behaviours, for example, are often placed alongside very vulnerable people, their needs for asylum taking precedence over the safety of more vulnerable people (Thompson and Brown 1998).

But while this acknowledgement is a step forward for individuals (see Brown 1994), the new discourse risks personalising forms of mistreatment that arise out of societal and structural inequalities. At an individual level, when issues of power are overlooked or neutralised, abusive and exploitative interactions can be explained away as relationships of choice. At a service level, new fault-lines between agencies, and between purchasers, providers and regulators set up contingencies that make abuse more likely and less visible. At a societal level, there is growing inequality between the pay and working conditions of managerial, professional and so-called 'unqualified' staff within and across the statutory, private (for-profit) and voluntary (not-for-profit) sectors. Gender and race exacerbate the unequal position of direct care staff and the disproportionate responsibility that falls on them.

The chapter divides into three parts. First, I shall review the current usage of the term 'abuse', looking at how it is being defined and categorised. Second, I will outline what is emerging as good practice in this field. Finally, I want to extend the debate to consider the impact of wider social inequalities, service structures and public policies as sources of abuse and mistreatment. When abuse of individuals is located in this broader context it is clear that adult protection practice needs to address both the personal and the political if it is to achieve and assure personal safety on behalf of *all* service users.

What is meant by the term 'abuse'?

When people say they do not know what abuse 'means' they are usually reflecting the very difficult ethical and professional judgements that need to be made when assessing risk and harm in the lives of adults whose autonomy as well as safety is an important issue. Consensus is beginning to emerge in relation to which *categories* of abuse should be covered within adult protection procedures. The Association of Directors of Social Services (ADSS) (1996) reflects this consensus by suggesting that all authorities should develop policies to cover:

*   physical abuse;
*   sexual abuse;
*   psychological abuse (sometimes called emotional or social abuse);
*   financial abuse;
*   neglect.

However, practitioners usually say that it is not the *category* but the *threshold of seriousness* (the point at which they should report their concerns) that they find difficult to pinpoint. They find this threshold particularly difficult to define in situations where a vulnerable adult is not asking for outside help but in which he or she might be being isolated, intimidated or exploited. Brown and Stein (1998) suggest a number of criteria to use in making this assessment, including individuals' frailty and their capacity to make decisions for themselves, the effect the abuse is having on them and on others, the likelihood of it being repeated or escalated and the risk of it extending to other vulnerable adults or children.

Where information has been gathered about *all* types of abuse it is evident that physical abuse predominates and frequently forms a component of other forms of abuse, such as sexual, financial or emotional abuse and neglect (see Kitson and Craft 1994; Brown and Stein 1998; Cambridge 1998). In cases of abuse reported under generic Adult Protection procedures in Kent and East Sussex (see Brown and Stein 1998) 135 people with learning disabilities were registered as having been abused within a twelve-month period. Of these, more than half (seventy cases) involved some kind of physical violence, twenty-one of which were compounded by other forms of abuse. People with learning disabilities across the whole age range were reported as victims of such abuse, with a peak of risk for young adults between 18 and 29. Both men and women were victims of physical violence. In many ways this mirrors the pattern of *sexual* abuse of people with learning disabilities (Brown, Stein and Turk 1995) except that in cases of sexual violence the perpetrators are predominantly men. The physical assaults were perpetrated by three main groups of people:

- by other service users in twelve cases;
- by staff in fifteen cases;
- by relatives in eleven cases.

In two cases the assaults were perpetrated by spouses, demonstrating the importance of making links, on behalf of people with learning disabilities, with generic abuse agencies, including those working to prevent and respond to domestic violence, racial harassment and broader community safety issues.

The physical abuse that was reported including hitting and rough handling; it was manifested as bruising, finger marks, lesions or burn marks. Over-medication or misuse of medical procedures may also fall within this category. Insensitive intimate care may result in harm, such as inept feeding or cleaning of teeth, while intrusive intimate care, for example the use of enemas without sound medical reasons or safeguards in their administration, may also be damaging. Lessons from inquiries (see for example Cambridge 1998; Wardhaugh and Wilding 1993; Buckinghamshire County Council 1998) suggest that physical abuse is more likely to occur in settings where care staff have little understanding of challenging behaviours, or assume that it is directed at them personally. This might result in individual reprisals but also in the more pervasive distortion of behavioural programmes, or 'sanctions', leading to serious and repeated assaults being carried out under the guise of punishment or control. An example is found in the complaint that Gordon Rowe punched a resident in the face for having defecated in bed (Buckinghamshire County Council 1998: 27), slapped another man who had wet himself on the sofa during an epileptic fit (1998: 44), and confined a resident to bed for a week because he did not want to work in the garden (1998: 28). Cambridge describes a regime in which care staff were told:

> the first hit was important. After the first hit, the person concerned would respect you and do as they were told. These

behaviours are typical of the ritualised disciplinary techniques associated with institutions.

(1998: 22)

Alternatively, more mundane physical hardships are imposed over a longer period, for example the exclusion of people who were late from meals (Buckinghamshire County Council 1998: 20 and 21). Other instances have been documented in which service users have been sent outside in all weathers because they have difficulty eating, or hosed down with cold water as a response to epilepsy or incontinence (Registered Homes Tribunal Decision 1991: 221; Buckinghamshire County Council 1998: 25). Guidance on the use (and non-use wherever possible) of restraint is urgently needed (see Harris *et al.* 1996), setting out a series of graduated interventions ensuring that the minimum of force is used to keep people safe.

Psychological abuse is often wrapped up in these situations but obscured because the mental health needs of people with learning disabilities are overlooked. Signs of mental distress tend to be explained away as part of the person's condition rather than as a valid emotional response to life events (Brown and Stein 1998). A recent research study on elder abuse unpacked this term to mean mainly verbal assault, threats and insults, including humiliation in relation to bodily functions such as incontinence and threats to abandon the vulnerable person (see Pillemer and Finkelhor 1988: 53, who term this 'chronic verbal aggression').

But although physical abuse is the most common form of harm recorded, recent concern has been more vocal in relation to sexual abuse. This reflects public outrage expressed about all sexual crimes at this time and not necessarily because these incidents are more serious than physical assaults and abuses. Pillemer and Finkelhor observe similar inconsistency in the field of elder abuse within which spouse abuse tends to have been downplayed in relation to abuse of older people by other persons, 'not due to the less serious nature of this abuse but instead to the more ambiguous moral imagery that this problem conjures up' (1988: 57). While physical abuse may be obscured or justified because of the 'difficulty' of managing people with learning disabilities or the necessity of being 'in control' or because the carer is 'under pressure', sexual abuse by a care worker or family member does not happen by accident or as a result of stress. Stress may indirectly lead to the use of alcohol or drugs that could act as disinhibitors but even then there is a shriller public outcry against sexual than other violent crimes. Sexual abuse is also unlikely to be a one-off occurrence, making it the most critical form of abuse when it comes to intervention. Although the judicial and quasi-judicial system often treat sexual offences as an isolated lapse, evidence from offenders suggests that their offences are often actively set up rather than triggered by specific situational factors (Waterhouse *et al.* 1994; Thompson and Brown 1998). Men with learning disabilities who commit sexual offences may also operate in this way but service workers often overlook serious sexual assaults when these are committed against other service users or women staff (Brown and Thompson 1997): they fail to organise timely interventions, leaving the men at risk of committing more high-profile crimes that risk leading to incarceration. Using definitions that focus consistently on harm to victims may help to clarify the need for intervention in such cases (Thompson and Brown 1998).

Definition is made more difficult because intimate care crosses usual boundaries and leaves both parties unsure where new lines can be drawn (Thompson *et al.* 1997). Same-sex care is still not specified in contracts and staff ratios are not calculated on the basis of gender. Training and support for staff often deals with the written and public aspects of the job but not with either the practicalities or feelings involved in toileting, menstrual management, masturbation and so on. Young inexperienced staff, or staff from backgrounds in which strict rules are applied to sexual matters are likely to be personally as well as professionally challenged by such tasks, but their invisibility and 'taboo' quality makes this difficult to address through the usual avenues of supervision or staff meetings. Where sexual issues are not addressed openly they tend to become the focus of innuendo or are driven underground into a prurient subculture in which abuse can flourish. Although research demonstrates that perpetrators of sexual (as opposed to other forms of) abuse are disproportionately men, women may also contribute to this kind of culture and/or it may leak into blurred boundaries or sexual harassment within the staff group.

A central issue when defining sexual abuse is to assess the person's ability to give informed and meaningful consent. Many services hide behind a rhetorical commitment to 'choice' that fails to discriminate between real choice and decisions foisted on, or made for, the person by staff or relatives. Any sexual behaviours, whether they involve direct contact or not, can be abusive in the absence of valid consent or in the presence of force or intimidation. These include non-contact abuse such as voyeurism, involvement in pornography, indecent exposure, harassment, serious teasing or innuendo, which may be experienced as particularly serious if they take place in a threatening atmosphere. In determining if someone can give consent there are three issues (Murphy and Clare 1995; Brown and Turk 1992):

- If the person *did* give their consent, because if they did not they have been raped or assaulted like any other woman or man.
- If the person *could* give their consent, that is if they understood enough about sexual behaviour and knew what was happening. In law, people with severe learning disabilities are deemed not to be able to give consent to sexual acts.
- A judgement has to be made as to whether the person with learning disabilities was *under undue pressure* in this particular situation, for example due to an authority or care-giving relationship, such as might be the case if sex is initiated by a staff or family member, or where force, trickery or exploitation are used. Physical force or the threat of violence or reprisals also cut across any meaningful consent.

The law specifies a distinction between people with severe intellectual impairments and those with milder degrees of disability; it is important that services undertake, or draw on, clear assessments of the capacity of individual service users who are engaging in sexual activities. When people with severe learning disabilities are sexually active, services should satisfy themselves that any sex they have is within mutual or reciprocal relationships and be prepared to advocate for them if this is challenged. When supporting people with mild learning difficulties, judgements hinge upon whether or not the relationships appear to have exploitative or threatening elements. Many chosen relationships contain elements of abuse and services have to make sensitive decisions about if or when to step in, for example if one person is misleading the other or if there is violence within the relationship (McCarthy and Thompson 1997).

Sexual abuse of people with learning disabilities takes place against a background of negative expectations about sex. People may have little in the way of credible or reliable sex education, have few opportunities to make friends or find privacy, and are always swimming against the tide if they wish to establish an independent sexual life (Brown 1994). Unfortunately, this kind of protective veneer does not keep people safe, merely ignorant. It means that they are often ill equipped to make a complaint, to appreciate when they might be putting themselves at risk or to have their problems picked up through routine health checks. Because workers often assume that people with learning disabilities are not sexually active, their sexual health needs tend not to be routinely addressed. They may not be offered smear tests, ordinary help with menstruation (as opposed to more drastic measures like hysterectomy) or safer-sex education.

Financial, or material, abuse is also an issue for people with learning disabilities, although one that is not often reported within the framework of abuse policies. Practitioners are often aware that people with learning disabilities have very restricted access to money and property. It is however striking that this does not lead to reports from staff or others in the way that more tangible or fraudulent transactions involving older people do (Brown and Stein 1998). Families may subsume benefits into the family income and irregularities in managing personal money in residential services are also commonplace (Bewley 1997). Professionals need to satisfy themselves about whether or not transactions or gifts are valid and uncoerced. Consent needs to be considered carefully as it does in relation to sexual interactions. Occasionally, formal measures are taken where individuals lack capacity but more often people make informal arrangements that are condoned by those around as long as they seem to work in the interests of the person concerned. The recent Green Paper (Law Commission 1997) specifies that proprietors of residential homes should not normally be appointees for the management of residents' personal finances, a situation that occurred in the Longcare homes (Buckinghamshire County Council 1998: 20). Other professionals may be aware of these arrangements and should be alert to problems, especially when the care provided is in other ways inadequate, or bordering on neglect. In the independent sector there is always a potential conflict of interest between profit and money spent on residents: one complainant at Longcare alleged that 'an insufficient portion of the income of Longcare Ltd was being spent on the residents' (Buckinghamshire County Council 1998: 26), so individual abuses may have corporate overtones.

Neglect would apply to situations within which an individual's basic physical, social and health care needs are not being met, for example failure to access proper medical or dental care, give prescribed medication or pain relief reliably or enable someone to use services such as a day centre or leisure group. Sometimes negligence is also included, implying a more active failure to take risks into account.

In cases involving all vulnerable adults reported under new adult protection policies in Kent and East Sussex during 1995–6, one-fifth of cases involved multiple forms of abuse within the same relationship. Hence, categorising 'acts' may not be as important as recognising the ongoing dynamics within bullying or exploitative relationships.

Bennett *et al.* (1997: 10) proposed a taxonomy that focuses on relationship and setting as opposed to type of harm. About half the reports made under the adult protection policies in Kent and East Sussex concerned people living in residential homes rather than individuals living in their own homes (Brown and Stein 1998). Problems in reporting make comparisons difficult and estimates of incidence incomplete: clearly many cases do not come to light and/or when they emerge single 'specimen' incidents are recorded instead of a retrospective catalogue of incidents. Cases are documented at different stages, at the initial 'alert' or referral, or later during an investigation or after a case conference. When the facts do emerge there is usually a consensus as to how serious the acts have been, but 'reading the runes' is more difficult. Lists of signs and symptoms of abuse are not based on thorough research or systematic observation. Practitioners are often urged to watch for 'changes' but often abuse is long-standing and/or worsens incrementally, so sudden changes are not evident. Many cases are not pursued because of lack of evidence even where significant concerns remain. Nevertheless, despite these methodological difficulties at a practice level, it is clear that it is the *identification* of abuse within the context of a number of more or less closed interlocking systems that is problematical rather than the definition.

Principles of good practice

'Adult protection' is beginning to be recognised as a distinct sphere of social work practice but one that is under-theorised and as yet under-developed: relevant skills such as investigative and interviewing skills, conflict resolution and mediation have yet to be developed in many authorities. At a theoretical level, abuse of children and vulnerable adults has been helpfully located within family dynamics (Kingston and Penhale 1995) and within institutional systems (Wardhaugh and Wilding 1993). Sobsey (1994) and Cambridge (1998) synthesise different approaches by stressing the links between individual interaction and both service and societal contexts, indicating a need for intervention at different levels and at different stages. Prevention, investigation, response and post-abuse support are all important but policies in the United Kingdom tend, like their counterparts in the US, to focus on case-finding and identification to the detriment of these issues (Daniels *et al.* 1989).

In terms of identification and investigation procedures, social services departments take the lead in cases involving vulnerable adults living at home because of their powers and duties under the NHS and

Community Care Act, 1990, while Inspection Units may take the lead in relation to specific concerns or allegations when the person lives in residential care, using powers set out in the Residential Homes Act, 1983. Where criminal prosecution is being considered the police may take charge and where disciplinary action is needed an employer must take the lead. This is fertile ground for crossed lines of communication and allocating someone to co-ordinate these parallel enquiries is a key issue at the start of any investigation (Brown *et al.* 1998). The Longcare inquiry asserts that:

> There have to be agreements on lead responsibilities, specific tasks, co-operation, communication and the best use of skill. Those inter-agency agreements must be in place so that they can be activated quickly when needed.
>
> (Buckinghamshire County Council 1998: 6)

It also advocates joint investigations within which:

> each agency moves forward with its task with maximum efficiency and taking advantage of the others' skills (for example joint interviews) with the knowledge that neither is prejudicing the other's inquiries or ability to act.
>
> (1998: 48)

When a vulnerable adult lacks 'capacity' to make decisions about the nature or extent of any enquiries, professionals have to act thoughtfully on their behalf. Matters of fact may be difficult to adjudicate and risks to other vulnerable adults may also have to be considered. It is largely because these judgements are so ethically complex that adult protection work depends on clear guidelines for communication, decision making and taking action, usually vested in a formal assessment or investigation followed by a case conference.

Focusing on identification and investigation is clearly an important place to start but not to finish. An adult protection strategy that focused on *prevention* would highlight, for example, rigorous screening at the recruitment stage, independent advocacy (Buckinghamshire County Council 1998: 24) and strong regulatory powers, but recent service development trends have been in the opposite direction, focusing on devolving responsibility for staffing to individual provider agencies, and working within a weak regulatory system. The registering authority has to prove someone unfit to be a proprietor or manager of a residential home rather than the opposite, as would be the case in a job interview. In theory, care management should provide a strong lever to ratchet up quality but this can only work where resources allow moderate case loads and where there is a choice of alternative placements. These issues are clearly salient but because they are structural they tend to have been treated as out of bounds, and energy has gone into drawing up a more limited adult protection strategy focused on investigation and immediate response. There is some evidence that these imbalances will be redressed with more focus on best value as opposed to compulsory competitive tendering, with a General Social Care Council and a stronger regulatory framework being mooted (Brand 1998; Burgner 1996).

An adult protection strategy that focused on *post-abuse support* would build up community-based networks, self-help groups and links with generic counselling and relief agencies, and develop skills in working with both abused and abusing people. There is evidence that such activity is feasible and some new services are being developed, for example a specialist counselling and assessment service for people with learning disabilities who have been sexually abused or are sexually abusing others (Respond), and a specialist refuge for women with learning disabilities (Beverley Lewis House) but these are both London-based. Practitioners may be sceptical about being mandated to report abuse when they know that a lack of appropriate service provision may make the situation worse, or lead to admission into more institutional forms of care (see Daniels *et al.* 1989, who describe this as a problem in the US).

Feeding knowledge from reported cases back into systems and service design and managing inter-agency relationships are both ongoing tasks suggesting the need for some kind of permanent review and co-ordinating body that may become known as an Adult Protection Committee, mirroring its counterparts in child protection. This would be a significant staging post in the development of adult protection work because it would provide a focal point for monitoring, learning and review.

Unfortunately, there is no coherent legislative provision in the United Kingdom for protecting the interests of vulnerable adults as there is for children. In some states in the US there are adult protection statutes that make it mandatory for anyone with concerns to report them to the authorities; bring together all agencies to draw up a plan for the person's protection and future support, and protect whistle-blowers. Many of the policies and procedures currently being introduced in the United Kingdom are designed to do the same job but without a coherent legal context. The fragmented nature of the legislative framework forms an unhelpful backdrop to the complex decisions that have to be made about how to protect the vulnerable person and what action to take against the individual responsible for the abuse. Most frame the abusive act as a matter of individual, rather than corporate, responsibility and frequently barriers to justice lead to informal and *ad hoc* sanctions, as the justice system proves impervious to people with learning disabilities and fails to accept their evidence. The need for reform has been acknowledged (Mencap 1997).

Adult protection in the context of new service structures

The focus on abuse as an isolated event or interaction, and its portrayal as a personal responsibility may mask the context within which it takes place and put too much emphasis on individuals rather than structures. Cambridge (1998), who describes a case of persistent abuse in a staffed house for two people with challenging behaviours, reports barriers to disclosure and reporting at all levels: for individuals (on account of communication difficulties); within the staffed house (because of threats and intimidation within the staff group); across the wider professional network (due to sporadic contact and lack of training in procedures related to abuse); and at the organisational level (because the contract was unclear about who should do what, equivocal in its support for whistle-blowers, naïve in its use of audit and inspection, and unclear about who should intervene once difficulties had been recognised). Brown and Thompson (1997) note similar confusion between purchaser and provider agencies about who is in charge, echoing Cambridge's observation that the mixed market has 'opened fractures in accountability' (1998: 25) that might not cause these situations but which allows them to flourish and certainly makes responding more clumsy and ineffective.

The recent independent inquiry into Longcare Ltd conducted for Buckinghamshire Social Services (1998), which documents abuse and mistreatment over a period of years in two homes for adults with learning disabilities yields further lessons. Obviously, the practice at these homes is not typical of other homes as it led to this high-profile inquiry, but nor can it be assumed to be an isolated example and similar situations are described in decisions of the Registered Homes Act Tribunal. For the purpose of this chapter it is cited as a test case – an exemplar not a representative case – and one that tested the system at various decision points. A superficial reading of the inquiry report is that is presents the 'bad apple' model of abuse and abusing, naming the proprietor of the home as the originator of much of the abuse and of the regime. But a more in-depth analysis shows the abuse to have been rooted in the dynamics of the establishment and its hierarchy, in its relationships with the outside world and in its position *vis-à-vis* public accountability within the contractual and regulatory processes set out in the NHS and Community Care Act of 1990. The report highlights a number of issues including:

- shortfalls in knowledge and skill among direct care staff;
- lack of appreciation of special needs in relation to difficult behaviour, sensory impairments and communication;
- splitting between professional and unqualified staff;
- the cumulative effect of social inequalities;
- conflicts between the development and policing role of purchasers and regulators.

A review of this and other recent cases (e.g. Cambridge 1998) suggests serious shortfalls in relevant skill and knowledge bases amongst people working directly with service users, specifically in residential settings. This leads hard-pressed staff to clutch at theoretical straws when it comes to their management of difficult residents. Oppressive regimes may then be bolstered by spurious theoretical claims that relatively untrained staff are not in a position to challenge, with the consequence that abuses are dressed up as some form of therapy. In the Longcare inquiry for example, a former member of staff made a complaint about the 'adversive [*sic*] behaviour modification techniques' in opera-tion in the regime, presumably referring to aversive techniques which are not currently advocated in professional circles (see Emerson *et al.* 1994 for an exposition of active support as an alternative strategy). Another witness described how a woman who did not like to sit and eat her meals at the dining table was made to sit in her chair in the dining room all day. This was described as a 'saturation technique' (Buckinghamshire County Council 1998: 64). Reference is made to 'privileges' being removed (having personal possessions confiscated). In a similar case, the hosing down of a young man with epilepsy was justified on the grounds that this was 'redirection therapy' (Registered Homes Tribunal 1993). As Stanley notes in Chapter 1, Frank Beck justified his regime with the term, 'regression therapy' (D'Arcy and Gosling 1998). These distortions could not have persisted if members of care staff had enough of a grounding to know that what they were witnessing was well outside the parameters of accepted practice.

This is the domain of psychologists but whereas there is a clear framework for professional accountability in the prescribing and control of medication, in the realm of teaching, learning and managing behaviour there are none. Psychologists are largely absent from residential care services; on the health side of the health/social-care divide they are not centrally involved in training or supervising social-care staff, or in shaping and policing *regimes*. They have no formal advisory role or management responsibility within the social-care system. So interventions are set in motion within homes that do not rest on any coherent understanding of behaviour and are not tested against any clear outcome measures. The blurring of professional/clinical expertise with lay models of care, based mostly on popular versions of child care (a resident at Longcare was sent to bed for being 'a naughty boy', Buckinghamshire County Council 1998: 41), has been a feature of so-called 'ordinary life' services.

The rhetoric of ordinariness has been a mixed blessing for people with learning disabilities. It has acted to reduce stigma and reduce distance between people with learning disabilities and the general public but it confuses issues around difference and impairment. Without knowledge of cognitive and sensory impairments or challenging behaviour, workers in services are left not knowing what to do when ordinary strategies fail to work. They are not helped to acquire knowledge that would allow them to empathise with the world as it is experienced by people with learning disabilities, to understand what individual service users take from verbal and other forms of communication or to tolerate their responses to difficulties and demands. If they were helped to enter into this *extra*ordinary world, difficult behaviour might not be seen as wilful and a justification for 'discipline' or 'sanctions', whether that be locking someone in their room, removing so-called 'privileges' from them or more actively 'punishing' them. A model is in operation whereby a lot of knowledge is held by a few people instead of one in which all staff are provided with a grounding across a number of academic disciplines, as is the case in Hungary and Italy where training in 'pedagogy' is seen as a requirement for all staff. Care work is designated outside of the scope of professional training, regulation and accountability presumably so that costs can be contained, but this creates a dangerous split.

If knowledge and expertise are not the keys to hierarchical power within care homes, then what is? The blurring of these establishments as homes and places of work create unacknowledged hierarchies in which some people labour under cumulative disadvantages while others are able to amplify their power and control over others. Gordon Rowe intimidated residents, staff and regulators alike in Longcare. He intimidated women using his power as a man and he intimidated men using his power as an employer. One of the first complainants waited to voice his concerns because he was waiting to be paid for work he had already done. His fears did not arise in a vacuum but were the result of a specific threat that 'if he reported concerns to anybody and the business failed he would be financially liable' (Buckinghamshire County Council 1998: 37). The inquiry report concludes that the whole regime 'might fairly be described as oppressive' and that 'It was an indication of the degree of control exercised by Gordon Rowe that respectable and responsible members of staff did not report the conditions of the homes to the Authority' (1998: 60).

The presence of married couples working in this sector also cuts across formal channels of accountability (see Registered Homes Tribunal 1991). In this service Gordon Rowe's deputy and co-director was his second wife, Angela Rowe, who was herself indicted for her part in the mistreatment of residents. Far from providing any checks or balances to the excesses of her husband she followed and bolstered his regime. It emerged at her trial that she had not read the code of practice, *Home Life* (Centre for Policy on Ageing 1984), despite being a co-director of the company. Another link was Ray Craddock, the manager of one of the Longcare homes, who was married to Gordon Rowe's first wife. Similarly, Decision 221 of the Registered Homes Tribunal (1993) documents abuse by the husband of the registered proprietor, a man who had no qualifications in care and no formal role within the home but who exerted considerable influence in the day-to-day dynamics of the household. The regulatory process is designed to scrutinise formal workplace relationships, not informal family-based dynamics, but it is the latter that often dominate in residential homes and small businesses. Acker (1990) observes that traditional theorising about organisations fails to recognise how:

> gendered attitudes and behaviour are brought into (and contaminate) essentially gender-neutral structures. This view of organisations separates structures from the people in them.
>
> (1990: 142)

This oversight is particularly inappropriate to situations where sexual abuse is alleged or uncovered, as theory 'which is blind to sexuality does not immediately offer avenues into the comprehension of gender domination' (1990: 140). Organisational theorists have pointed to the extent to which management theory and practice rests on assumptions about masculinity (Hearn and Parkin 1987). In the case of residential homes there is a need to challenge not only the way male power is used within the employer–employee relationship but within the living situation and social relations of the home, particularly the assumption that the use of male power as a form of authority is a legitimate therapeutic strategy.

Nor should gender dynamics be seen only in relation to personal alliances or to the dominance of men over women (whether married to them or their employers), since male power is also cemented through membership of such organisations as the Freemasons, as noted in the Longcare case (Buckinghamshire County Council 1998: 9). The Longcare report states that Gordon Rowe's claims to 'have a good relationship with the police were taken as a threat' (Buckinghamshire County Council 1998: 41). Masonic influence has been suggested as a factor in relation to other high-profile cases (D'Arcy and Gosling 1998: 62). Unions have also been implicated but these are not the only collectives to have been unwittingly drawn into collusion with abusers in this way. Both Frank Beck and Mark Trotter courted their local political parties (Liberal and Labour respectively) to provide a power base from which to carry on their activities (D'Arcy and Gosling 1998: 68). Acker and Van Houten argue that *'sex power differentials outside the organisation act as a power multiplier enhancing the authority of male superiors in the workplace'* (1992: 18), so that when analysing regimes it is important to register these extraneous forms of power. This indeed presents a whole set of problems for regulators and commissioners. A formal and impartial regulatory structure has to act as if these relationships and alliances do not exist when they may be critical in underpinning ongoing abuses of power and masterminding resistance to legitimate challenges.

In terms of accountability there is still work to be done concerning the balance between purchasers, regulators and providers of care. The newly commercialised context sets up complicated dynamics (ARC/NAPSAC 1993) that make open acknowledgement of abuse risky for providers operating within a commercial context. It is easy to see how they could be influenced to keep abusive incidents hidden or allow a perpetrator to resign in a way that leaves him or her in a position to work with vulnerable adults again. Alternatively, some of these situations come about because cost-cutting on the part of purchasers has led to service providers being unable to provide the level of service specified in a worthy but unworkable contract. Several placing authorities may be involved in a situation in which a lead is being taken by another authority's regulatory body, resulting in difficult decisions about how to co-ordinate and when to release information. There may be role confusion between care managers (responsible for monitoring the quality of an individual placement) and inspectors (responsible for monitoring the quality of a whole establishment) such as those that led the Longcare inquiry to remark that 'responsible social workers and Inspectors do not play on opposing teams' (Buckinghamshire County Council 1998).

Nor is the regulatory relationship straightforward: it hinges on whether purchasers and regulators should deal with these issues in an open and transparent style or conduct more covert and underhand investigations in order to maintain more proactive 'intelligence' on care providers and agencies. Sir William Utting (1991) identified this tension at the beginning of the development of the new arm's length inspection and regulatory structures, distinguishing between inspection as 'regulation' and inspection as 'development'. He highlighted the incompatibility between 'a legalistic approach and a more advisory, supportive role' that was echoed in the more recent Longcare inquiry (Buckinghamshire County Council 1998). This duality is particularly apparent in relation to sexual or financial abuse, which are usually covert and easily covered up during scheduled inspections or audits.

Regulation takes place against the background of these contradictory dynamics and seeks to assume a quasi-management role, not only setting standards but helping to identify resources and encourage staff training while at the same time having a policing and enforcement role. Matters that would have been dealt with as routine management issues within a local authority or other publicly funded service structure are now aired and tested in the quasi-legal arena of the Tribunal. Intermediate options such as moving staff, monitoring or supervising them more closely, reassigning them to work that does not place service users at risk and so on are no longer available options. Closure decisions are also made more difficult because of the problem of disruption to residents, leading to a request for clarification in the Longcare inquiry about who should manage homes in the immediate aftermath of an emergency closure by magistrate's order. On the other hand, it must be noted that public monopolies also failed to recognise and act in the face of similar abuse such as that perpetrated by Frank Beck (D'Arcy and Gosling 1998). The Longcare inquiry resolved this tension by asserting that the 'policing' role should take precedence over the 'advisory' role (Buckinghamshire County Council 1998: 24) but this begs the question of who then acts in this advisory capacity given the dearth of relevant knowledge and training in some (but by no means all) homes.

Conclusion

While the discourse of abuse recognises individual people with learning disabilities as victims and begins a process whereby they may be supported in seeking justice and redress, abuse also needs to be acknowledged as a product of structural inequalities and 'fractures of accountability' (Cambridge 1998). The abuse at Longcare occurred in a dynamic force-field at the meeting point of unchecked male power, poorly trained and ill-supported staff, conflicts between a profit and care ethic and weak 'arm's length' regulation. The parameters of the new adult protection policies have been shaped in response to this 'market' context but while they encourage individual workers to report abuse, and regulators to be alert to signals of inadequate or oppressive regimes, there are wider structural issues that they do not and cannot touch. Workers in abusive regimes are often underpaid, untrained and insecure; they may be afraid of the proprietor, management or union and be unable to 'blow the whistle' (see Pilgrim 1995 and Wardhaugh and Wilding 1993). These personal inequalities reflect a new set of economic relationships in the care 'industry' that need to be taken into account if adult protection work on behalf of people with learning disabilities is to be effective and robust.

References

Acker, J. (1990) 'Hierarchies, jobs, bodies: A theory of gendered organisations', *Gender and Society* 4: 139–58.

Acker, J. and Van Houten, D. (1992) 'Differential recruitment and control', in A. Mills and P. Tancred (eds) *Gendering Organizational Analysis*, London: Sage.

ADSS (1966) *Resolution on Adult Protection Policies*, Association of Directors of Social Services c/o Knowsley Social Services.

ARC/NAPSAC (eds) (1993) *It Could Never Happen Here: The Prevention and Treatment of Sexual Abuse of Adults with Learning Disabilities in Residential Settings*, Nottingham: NAPSAC.

Barron, D. (1996) *A Price to be Born*, Harrogate: Mencap Northern Division.

Bennett, G., Kingston, P. and Penhale, B. (eds) (1997) *The Dimensions of Elder Abuse*, Basingstoke: Macmillan.

Bewley, C. (1997) *Money Matters*, London: Values into Action.

Brand, D. (1998) 'Commentary on adult abuse issues', *Tizard Learning Disability Review* 3(1): 27–30.

Brown, H. (1994) 'An ordinary sexual life?: A review of the normalisation principle as it applies to the sexual options of people with learning disabilities', *Disability and Society* 9(2): 123–44.

Brown, H., Brammer, A., Craft, A. and McKay, C. (1996) *Towards Better Safeguards: A Handbook on the Sexual Abuse of Adults with Learning Disabilities for Inspection and Registration Officers*, Brighton: Pavilion Publishing.

Brown, H., Skinner, R., Stein, J. and Wilson, B. (1998) *The Investigator's Guide: The AIMS Series*, Brighton: Pavilion Publishing.

Brown, H. and Stein, J. (1998) 'Implementing adult protection policies in Kent and East Sussex', *Journal of Social Policy* 27(3): 371–96.

Brown, H., Stein, J. and Turk, V. (1995) 'The sexual abuse of adults with learning disabilities: Report of a second two year incidence survey', *Mental Handicap Research* 8(1): 3–24.

Brown, H. and Thompson, D. (1997) 'Service responses to men with intellectual disabilities who have sexually abusive or unacceptable behaviours: The case against inaction', *Journal of Applied Research in Intellectual Disability* 10(2): 176–97.

Brown, H. and Turk, V. (1992) 'Defining sexual abuse as it affects adults with learning disabilities', *Mental Handicap* 20(2): 44–55.

Buckinghamshire County Council (1998) *Independent Longcare Inquiry*, Buckingham: Buckinghamshire County Council.

Burgner, T. (1996) *The Regulation and Inspection of Social Services*, London: Department of Health and Welsh Office.

Cambridge, P. (1998) 'The physical abuse of people with learning disabilities and challenging behaviours: Lessons for commissioners and providers', *Tizard Learning Disability Review* 3(1) 18–27.

Campbell, V., Smith, R. and Wool, R. (1982) 'Adaptive behaviour scale differences in scores of mentally retarded individuals referred for institutionalisation and those never referred', *American Journal of Mental Deficiency* 86(4): 425–8.

Carpenter, M. (1994) *Normality is Hard Work: Trade Unions and the Politics of Community Care*, London: Lawrence & Wishart with Unison.

Centre for Policy on Ageing (1984) *Home Life: A Code of Practice for Residential Care*, London: Centre for Policy on Ageing.

Daniels, R., Baumhover, L. and Clark-Daniels, C. (1989) 'Physicians' mandatory reporting of elder abuse', *The Gerontologist* 29(3): 321–7.

D'Arcy, M. and Gosling, P. (1998) *Abuse of Trust: Frank Beck and the Leicestershire Children's Homes Scandal*, London: Bowerdean Publishing Company.

Emerson, E., McGill, P. and Mansell, J. (eds) (1994) *Severe Learning Disabilities and Challenging Behaviours: Designing High Quality Services*, London: Chapman Hall.

Goffman, E. (1961) *Asylums*, Harmondsworth: Penguin.

Harris, J., Allen, D., Cornick, M. and Mills, R. (1996) *Physical Interventions: A Policy Framework*, Kidderminster: British Institute of Learning Disabilities.

Hearn, G. and Parkin, W. (1987) *'Sex at Work': The Power and Paradox of Organisation Sexuality*, Brighton: Wheatsheaf.

Jupp, K. (1991) *Seeking the Answers for those People with Learning Disabilities who Sexually Offend*, Kidderminster: British Institute of Mental Handicap.

Kingston, P. and Penhale, B. (eds) (1995) *Family Violence and the Caring Professions*, Basingstoke: Macmillan.

Kitson, D. and Craft, A. (1994) 'Green light for guidelines', *Community Care*, 7 April: 28–9.

Law Commission (1997) *Who Decides? Making Decisions on Behalf of Mentally Incapacitated Adults*, London: Lord Chancellor's Department, HMSO.

McCarthy, M. and Thompson, D. (1997) 'A prevalence study of sexual abuse of adults with intellectual disabilities referred for sex education', *Journal of Applied Research in Intellectual Disabilities* 10(2): 105–24.

Mencap (1997) *Barriers to Justice*, London: Mencap.

Murphy, G. and Clare, I.C.H. (1995) 'Adults' capacity to make decisions affecting the person: Psychologists' contribution', in R. Bull and D. Carson (eds) *Handbook of Psychology in Legal Contexts*, Chichester: Wiley.

Pilgrim, D. (1995) 'Explaining abuse and inadequate care', in G. Hunt (ed.) *Whistleblowing in the Health Service: Accountability, Law and Professional Practice*, London: Arnold.

Pillemer, K. and Finkelhor, P. (1988) 'The prevalence of elder abuse: A random sample survey', *The Gerontologist* 28(1): 51–7.

Registered Homes Tribunal (1991) Decision 162, West Sussex County Council.

—— (1993) Decision 221, Powys County Council.

Sobsey, R. (1994) *Violence and Abuse in the Lives of People with Disabilities*, Baltimore: Paul Brookes.

Stein, J. and Brown, H. (eds) (1996) *A Nightmare … That I Thought Would Never End: A Tape about Sexual Abuse for Staff Made by Service Users*, Brighton: Pavilion Publishing.

Thompson, D. and Brown, H. (1998) *Response-ability*, Brighton: Pavilion Publishing.

Thompson, D., Clare, I. and Brown, H. (1997) 'Not such an "ordinary" relationship: The role of women support staff in relation to men with learning disabilities who have difficult sexual behaviour', *Disability and Society* 12(4): 573–92.

Utting, W. (1991) *Children in the Public Care*, London: HMSO.

Wardhaugh, J. and Wilding, P. (1993) 'Towards an explanation of the corruption of care', *Critical Social Policy* 37: 4–31.

Waterhouse, L., Dobash, R.P. and Carnie, J. (1994) *Child Sexual Abusers*, Edinburgh: The Scottish Office Central Research Unit.

Williams, C. (1993) 'Vulnerable victims? A current awareness of the victimisation of people with learning disabilities', *Disability, Handicap and Society* 8(2): 161–72.

Wolfensberger, W. (1975) *The Origin and Nature of our Institutional Models: The Principle of Normalization in Human Services*, Toronto: Syracuse Human Policy Press.

—— (1980) 'The definition of normalization – update, problems, disagreements and misunderstandings', in R. Flynn and K. Nitsch (eds) *Normalization, Integration and Community Services*, Austin, Texas: Pro-ed.

5   Users' perceptions

Searching for the views of users with learning disabilities

Jill Manthorpe

> It used to make me laugh at The Park. They were so deceitful at the Park. Why couldn't they have told the truth when they used to have the Board of Control that came round every year. Well, they used to get all bathrooms and put towels on baths. Well, we never had towels. And they used to put soap in sinks. We never even saw soap! They did all that, just to make an impression. Anyway, I told 'em about it. I said 'You know it's not always like this, it's only because you've come.'
>
> Grace, quoted in Potts and Fido (1991: 23)

An atmosphere of anxiety pervades much institutional care for people with learning disabilities. Its evolution from hospital care (Atkinson 1988: 127) may account for the survival of certain traditions and practices associated with hospital life, but people with learning disabilities are increasingly reported as critical of features such as routine or over-organised domestic life (Mental Health Foundation: 1996). More fundamental, however, are their questions about the purpose of residential provision when policy emphasis is on community provision. We are currently witnessing, after the closure of the majority of long-stay hospitals specialising in mental handicap, a new pattern of entry to residential care. Rather than residential care being perceived as a less restrictive alternative to hospital (of course, not invariably so), entry to residential care is becoming a consequence of 'failed' community living or breakdowns in support. Those who cannot be maintained in the community on their own or with their family will be considered for residential care. This is contrary, of course, to the optimism inherent in the Wagner report (1988) that it could form part of a system of positive decision-making or choice, but more in line with financial realities restricting options.

The context of residential care for people with learning disabilities has changed immensely since the publication of the Wagner report and its accompanying background research papers. As Malin reports (1997), the majority of provision in residential care for people with learning disabilities is located in the independent and commercial sector of care.

However, the size and type of residential care now provided encompass significant variations: while large and highly staffed units exist, there are also units with minimal staffing such as group homes. It is clear that none are immune from abusive practices: Cambridge's (1998) report of abuse occurring in a small group home for two individuals reveals the vulnerability of such a setting, despite its efforts to be synonymous with a 'home', not an institution.

In this chapter we shall explore the views of people with learning disabilities about abuse in institutions. The first section takes a fresh look at the early influential inquiries into long-stay mental handicap hospitals to establish if patients' perspectives were included in this process of uncovering abuse. We then move to the small number of personal testimonies currently emerging, some produced by individuals themselves but publicised in the professional literature, others coming directly from research activity. The next section explores residents' perspectives from a recent inquiry into institutional abuse. Finally, we discuss individuals' experiences and those of their families, looking at attempts to raise issues publicly and also to provide protection and assistance to survivors.

Past inquiries – silent patients

Any work with people who have learning disabilities needs to take into account its context, and hospital provision has formed a dominant and long-standing backcloth to care. The creation of mental handicap hospitals, which for many decades were integrated with hospitals for people with mental illnesses, fulfilled multiple purposes – segregation, protection, care and control. These aims have been criticised both specifically and generally, for hospitals stand 'condemned as incapable of providing a good quality of life for people with learning difficulties' (Corkish and Heyman 1998: 217). Many of the characteristics of abusive behaviour have been identified in such hospital regimes: aspects of neglect, over-medication, physical ill-treatment and impersonal, poor-quality care. Recent years have witnessed the opportunity for former patients to describe at last their lives, but past inquiries are remarkable for their lack of attention to the patient perspective.

The report presented by the Committee of Inquiry into Allegations of Ill-Treatment of Patients and other Irregularities at the Ely

Hospital, Cardiff (1969), for example, is a highly detailed account of abuse that was initially drawn to public attention by a nursing assistant through the media. His allegations covered a wide variety of poor practices: cruelty and ill-treatment, general inhumane and threatening behaviour, pilfering of patients' and hospital belongings, indifference to complaints and a lack of care by the physician superintendent. As Martin notes, the significance of this inquiry was that it was thorough: it sought and found hard evidence. While the report found 'individual callousness, and sometimes brutality' (1984: 8) the system itself was perceived as deeply flawed.

Reading such reports now, the perspective of patients is hard to determine. It is clear that in the hospitals under scrutiny many staff felt intimidated and were unwilling to complain. In Ely, staff were further demoralised by inadequate supervision, scant training and victimisation. Such inquiries are useful in allowing junior staff to voice their concerns, both in relation to patient treatment and also in respect of their own roles. It is possible to link poor treatment of staff with abuse of patients, for it was the testimony of staff that enabled inquiries to acquire semi-objective knowledge of patient care. However, the disabilities and communication problems of the patients were deemed to be so extensive that evidence from them was not sought. The views of Ely's patients are missing.

This is not to portray all inquiries as objectifying patients, but this omission is a consequence of the then limitations of communication skills and attitudes of the time. The Farleigh inquiry (Committee of Inquiry into Farleigh Hospital 1971) is fairly typical in its attention to the difficulty of looking after the 'severely handicapped' who 'possess the bodies of grown men and the minds of small children' (1971: 1). The violence and ill-treatment meted out to patients was significantly targeted on those in an isolated ward with the most profound handicaps and difficult behaviours. None were deemed to be in a position to give evidence or effectively complain.

Such inquiries illustrate the problem of determining patients' perspectives; we are largely reliant on staff and these accounts were often contradicted by each other or open to interpretation. Patients' relatives, on occasion, were witness to abuses and the role played by Mr S.'s mother in the South Ockenden Hospital inquiry (Committee of Inquiry into South Ockenden Hospital 1974) is unusual but significant as she felt able to challenge hospital staff, though not without probably worsening her son's situation in the short-term and laying herself open to accusations of mental disturbance.

Similarly, in Normansfield Hospital (Committee of Inquiry into

Normansfield Hospital 1978) some patients' relatives were regular visitors to the wards and were able to identify that all was not well. In this inquiry considerable attention was given to individual patients, particularly to the questions of their medication and physical condition, in an attempt to explore the medical consultant's prescribing practices and exercise of control. Non-nursing staff, such as the teacher, were especially valuable in presenting a perspective from outside the culture of the health service with its hierarchy of doctor–nurse relationships. Furthermore, this inquiry reveals the potential of groups who are primarily interested in patients' welfare, rather than hospital functioning, namely the League of Friends. Their evidence provided the inquiry with a picture of changes and deterioration among patients and among hospital practices over time and illustrated the potential for those with commitment to patient well-being to contribute to the monitoring of quality.

Patient testimony

It is of course very difficult for anyone to make a complaint when the cost of doing so may be considerable. The accounts of abuse from people with learning disabilities tend to appear later in their lives. There is now some evidence as to their perceptions of institutional life – derived from the few personal testimonies that have only recently been circulated through publication. David Barron's life represents such an example (Barron 1987) while other accounts have been articulated through oral history projects and reminiscence work.

Barron describes his admission to Whixley in 1939, a mental deficiency institution near York, in harrowing detail. Aged 14, he was taken on his first day to a locked ward and locked into a bedroom at night:

> I learned later, I was in the punishment ward. It was an institutional ruling that you spent the first few months there. You weren't allowed to speak to other patients; all possessions were taken away; we were on half rations; a discipline of hard physical labour like scrubbing concrete with a brick and half a bucket of cold water.
>
> (1987: 8)

Barron's description almost defies contemporary attempts to classify abuse and evokes a real sense of the nature of institutional life with its inflexible routines and dehumanising practices. From his account the unfairness of incarceration comes to the fore, as well as the scope for some individuals in authority to exercise this kindly or abusively. In an institution founded on legal frameworks the discretion for staff to act according to their own moral codes appears extensive; abuse is here constructed as punishment – justifiable to ensure the smooth running of the organisation by emphasising the power hierarchy.

Barron's autobiography has been augmented by other sources, such as oral history and the investigation of documents or records. As Walmsley (1997) notes, oral testimonies stand in stark contrast to most official reports, but the accounts of people with learning disabilities are less accessible. The emphasis in oral history on finding people who are articulate (Walmsley 1997) may mean that people with communication difficulties or behavioural problems are left out of the search for those with 'a good story to tell'.

Interviews may help those who feel uncomfortable in telling their story and Fido and Potts (1997) succeeded in their work by talking to former hospital residents, some of whom had severe speech difficulties. It is clear from their reflections on this research that Fido and Potts believe that individual memories were often selective in the attempt to cope with feelings of acute distress and deprivation. Nonetheless, the interview material they obtained again paints a picture of tyrannical systems of institutional life, with emphasis on punishment as the key means of control. Punishment was built into the official rules of the hospital and into its physical fabric through the creation of punishment rooms, wards and villas. If we label such practices as abusive we challenge the whole edifice; if we label only 'extremes' as abuse we may accept what may be the unacceptable. The theme of punishment is not confined to users' experiences in mental handicap hospitals (it is noticeably missing from most professional and official reports of hospital life) but can be found in other guises. Reynolds refers to a system of behaviour modification that she found abusive in relation to a student she worked with who was being considered for a community placement. Reynolds puts herself in her student's (Jan's) shoes when presented with a sheet of responses that everyone was to make to Jan to change her behaviour:

> Everyone who was part of Jan's life was to respond on these lines. Saying these same words to her in response. It occurred to me that a case could be made out for this being a subtle form of torture. How would I feel if everyone I came into contact with suddenly changed their many and varied responses to me and all said the same things? If I was further told that this was how it was normal

to behave and I was not to be released from this situation until I also conformed to this pattern of response?

(1989: 30)

Reynolds also includes the experience of Albert, a member of a self-advocacy group who lived in a hostel and was labelled as having 'personality problems' (1989: 32). These stemmed from his objection to staff 'reasonably' chastising his girlfriend. The language of chastisement for an adult sits uncomfortably with the status of adulthood and emphasises again a point made in debates about ordinary living that people with learning disabilities are frequently infantilised. In institutions the power differentials between staff and residents can mirror the dynamics of a patriarchal family with residents being perceived as children, who are labelled 'naughty' when they make demands on staff and challenge their authority.

Listening to individuals' voices, however, reminds us further that abuse is often subjective. Mabel Cooper, for example, while outlining the poor conditions and treatment in her years in hospital, comments: 'They shouldn't put people what's been in a long-stay hospital on their own. I think that's the worst cruelty ever' (1997: 34).

As Atkinson (1994) comments on her reminiscence work with people with learning disabilities, stories of humour and defiance may emerge in discussions of hospital life, but she also identifies a distinction between public and private accounts. Both can contain painful memories but public accounts have been told many times and this repetition may have made the pain recede. She considers more private accounts that had not been shared and these had the capacity to be upsetting.

This work points to the value of personal testimony and the potential for it to influence perceptions of service development and professional practice. It also identifies the users' perspectives as complex and embedded in other narratives. Accounts of past abuses located in former institutions can run the risk of creating professional complacency about current practices.

In addition to the personal testimony, research studies provide some clues as to the broader experience of institutional life and help to forestall criticism that accounts such as Barron's are exceptional. Booth, Simons and Booth's (1990) research is valuable in this respect, for it collected the views of people with learning disabilities at intervals before their moves from hospital or hostel, immediately after the move and one year later. The researchers found that, prior to their move, most respondents were 'notably uncritical' of their environment (1990:

130). After their moves or relocation, the researchers discovered that respondents were expressing more negative comments about the hospital and hostels where they formerly lived. These included complaints about the atmosphere and their experiences of violence. New grievances were mentioned that had not been raised prior to the move. There were also fewer positive comments about their previous institutional homes.

The interviews conducted a year after the move showed a striking change, for respondents now made increasing reference to the stressful atmosphere of their previous homes and some were prepared to criticise individual staff: 'Many of our respondents reported distressing instances of assault and harassment by other residents and, in a few cases, by staff and outsiders' (1990: 141). As the researchers comment, hospital and hostel residents appeared to have had 'very low expectations' and: 'To many of them the nature of the institution was given; their adaptation to it was largely unquestioning. Things happened the way they did because that's the way they happen; if staff say it's good then it must be good' (1990: 140). Such research permits us to hear the views of residents and to develop the understanding that people with learning disabilities may be cautious in expressing criticism.

Resident perspectives

In the decades since these early inquiries there has been a continuing decrease in hospital numbers, although it is estimated that 11,400 people with learning disabilities are still resident in long-stay hospitals in the UK (Malin 1997: 133). Ramcharan (1998) warns that issues of abuse and quality of care remain in such settings, particularly in relation to those with the most severe disabilities. He identifies problems 'at the cusp of abuse' – infringements of residents' rights, questionable practices around seclusion, or entrenched behaviour and cultural patterns. While there exist policies in respect of abuse, these 'minor' problems do not seem to staff to warrant the perceived heavy hand of abuse policies, so the problems are left unresolved.

Such debates point to the central role of staff in responding to each others' behaviour. Despite enthusiasm and acclaim for independent representation, independent advocates remain infrequent and patchy visitors to institutions, mainly because there is no legislative requirement in force and because advocacy is not given priority by funding agencies. The report of the Law Commission (1995), *Mental Incapacity*, exposes the vulnerability of people who have no agreed mechanism for representation or decision-making and proposes a substitute decision-maker to be appointed by the judicial system. It is not clear to what extent such individuals will conceive their role as advocacy, but the potential for this function is evident.

Whilst past inquiries failed to identify the patient's voice as relevant, contemporary inquiries have developed some mechanisms for communication. The Longcare inquiry deserves to be seen as a major inquiry, of national significance, one which can be compared to those inquiries into hospitals reported above. As Hilary Brown has discussed in Chapter 4, the Longcare Inquiry (Buckinghamshire County Council 1998) was a 'test case' in some respects, primarily testing systems of regulation. This report does show evidence of direct communication between residents and certain staff with responsibility for the quality and provision of their care. For example, a social worker had reported to the Registration Officer concerns resulting from a conversation with a resident (at a relative's home) about Gordon Rowe's physical treatment of her and the observation of her injuries. The Registration Officer later interviewed this resident and others, and material arising from this complaint and further allegations formed the basis of grounds for improvement noted in the Annual Inspection Report. The inquiry observes that neither the resident nor her social worker were informed of the investigation; however, it comments that the resident could have been called to give evidence (there were no charges in this respect because of Rowe's death) and that 'she was regarded as competent to take oath and to give material evidence' (Buckinghamshire County Council 1998: 22).

Further contrast with the hospital inquiries can be seen in the direct submissions to the Longcare inquiry made on behalf of residents, parents and relatives. Indeed, an organisation, Justice for Longcare Survivors, was formed and helped elicit residents' views as well as campaigning for the inquiry report to be made public. The inquiry members visited the remaining residents and spoke to them in the presence of parents or social workers.

The residents' submissions to the inquiry cover three main areas, although residents' words are not reported directly. They observe that:

1 The parents, guardians and relatives ... have been left without information by the Authority and had experienced a great deal of pain and suffering.
2 The Authority had insufficient understanding of the damage done to Longcare residents or they would not have left the homes open and the current residents in place.

3   The fact that there is no criminal prosecution, or that a criminal prosecution is not successful, does not mean that the allegations are trivial. The criminal law standard of proof has to be high but it is not the test of fitness to be concerned in the running of residential homes for vulnerable people.

(Buckinghamshire County Council 1998: 83)

Brief details of six families' concerns are also appended to the inquiry as Appendix 4.

The Longcare inquiry recommends that the local authority invests in advocacy schemes to provide a means of reducing the incidence of abuse through increased self-confidence and the ability to prevent or minimise its effects. Advocacy, it also argues, should be available to provide counselling and support for victims of abuse and to assist individuals in raising issues or making complaints. The extent to which advocacy schemes are able to fulfil such expectations will have to be borne out in practice; advocacy has its advantages but its focus can be very general – quite rightly relating to what service users perceive as important.

The importance of listening to users' views of abuse is bound up with debates about users' influence over services and their lives in general. People with learning disabilities may have profound communication difficulties and hearing their 'voice' is not a simple process. It seems likely that advances in communication skills among practitioners will produce further allegations of abuse, as people are now able to express themselves more explicitly. Other developments may well occur at the time of the closure or transfer of long-stay hospital provision and the spotlight that can fall on patients at such times in relation to assessment and attempts to discern their wishes or preferences. Therapeutic work can also enable silent voices to be heard and can offer explanations as to why institutional dynamics may provide abusers with scope for exploitation. Sinason (1994), for example, details her therapeutic work making direct use of Miss Kay's description of horrific sexual abuse she experienced from a male instructor at an Adult Training Centre. Miss Kay was able to recount how the instructor had told her not to make a noise or her mother would die. With hindsight, Miss Kay's mother was able to identify how this could have happened within the centre. Sinason reports:

Mrs Kay believed her daughter completely. She could see how her distressed behaviour and emotional deterioration had led to outbursts at the Centre where the instructor was gratefully seen as a disciplinary aid in removing her from the large group. No-one considered anything that happened unusual. Because Miss Kay's behaviour was only seen in terms of an inability to settle in, her increased emotional disturbance was ignored. Each time she was removed from the room by this worker other staff were grateful.

(1994: 165)

The testimonies of survivors of abuse have so far failed to encompass people with learning disabilities from ethnic minority groups. In view of the over-representation of ethnic minority populations among young people with learning disabilities (Azmi *et al.* 1996) it will be increasingly important for practitioners to be able to respond to allegations of abuse that touch on cultural and religious matters. While Millard (1994), for example, reports on work with a group of women who constructed their own role play scenario to develop their assertiveness skills, she only briefly notes the relevance of ethnicity to the group's composition and functioning. In this women's group the initial focus was on sex education, but group members developed dramatic representations of abuse, bullying and discrimination. From such work it would appear that abuse within institutions is a very extensive 'blanket term' particularly when it obscures the level and nature of abuse. The women in this group, for example, raise matters concerning fellow male residents' behaviour, sexual harassment at work and unhelpful treatment by officials. A central theme of power and powerlessness unites all three.

Further experiences await expression in ways that can imbue communication with dignity and respect. These include experiences around other forms of abuse, besides sexual abuse, that, as Hilary Brown observes, is a dominant motif. This focus is particularly individualistic – an abuser is at fault and (generally) his exclusion will restore equilibrium to the individual and institution. Other forms of abuse exist in a 'grey' area where it is not so clear whether the individual is responsible or culpable or the institution creates and sustains an abusive culture. The Longcare inquiry (Buckinghamshire County Council: 1998) concentrates more on the individual power of Gordon Rowe and its perversity rather than questioning institutional life.

Perspectives on financial abuse

In contrast to sexual abuse, financial abuse is evidently easier for people to talk about – at least in some circumstances. Bewley's (1997) report, *Money Matters*, includes a range of stories told by individuals with learning disabilities:

> Many individuals with learning difficulties have a lot to say about their money. ... With support and encouragement people wanted to share their views and experiences. ... I was not just looking for bad stories; I wanted to hear about what was good, too. But I was surprised at the level of bad experiences people told me about. I did not have to dig at, or highlight, these stories; they were there on the surface.
>
> (1997: 10)

There may be a number of reasons for people's willingness to talk about money. To begin with, being the victim of financial abuse may not be as personally threatening to the health and safety of an individual as is sexual crime or abuse. It is an experience relatively common in the form of burglary or car crime and such victims' accounts are frequently reported in the media. It can and is seen to 'happen to anyone', although this may be a generalisation. Sexual abuse may evoke responses that are extreme, such as medical examination, accusations of confabulation and further personal and family distress. Financial abuse can of course be accompanied by other forms of abuse (multiple abuse) but can also be a 'fact of life' and at differing levels of seriousness.

Bewley's collection of the views of individuals with learning disabilities draws attention to possible abuse within institutional life. For example:

> In one place, home to about sixty women with learning difficulties, residents followed an old practice of queuing up every Saturday morning to receive £5 pocket money. Where the rest of their £14.10 personal allowance went was unclear. Certainly none of the residents knew that they might be entitled to at least twice the weekly amount they received.
>
> (1997: 480)

In another example, Alan and Tom explain how they had looked forward to receiving their own benefit income and opening their own bank accounts when they moved from a long-stay hospital to a group home, but their assets were frozen and for two years they have had to return to the hospital to access their own funds:

Every week, Alan and Tom have to make the long bus journey back to the place they never wanted to set eyes on again to get money from the hospital bank. ... Apart from being expensive and time consuming for them, and apart from the fact that it prevents them properly settling in their new homes and opening local bank accounts, it also causes great distress to the men, who have to walk back up the long drive and enter a place they hate and fear.

(1997: 13)

This example draws attention to the system of financial controls that many criticise as unwieldy and inappropriate for life outside hospital, where capacity is to be encouraged rather than removed. While this example may not constitute financial abuse by a person in a position of trust who deprives an individual of their money, it does constitute a denial of choice and opportunity. Clearly, to people with learning disabilities this matters.

Prevention and protection

Williams' (1995) influential report and training material on crime and abuse against people with learning disabilities places high value on techniques and strategies for prevention. Moreover, he argues that the best way to learn about prevention is to engage with 'personal experiences' of people with learning disabilities (1995: 43). These can include avoidance strategies such as minimising the insignia of disability around the physical appearance of buildings or individual safety programmes involving the diffusion of threatening incidents. He cautions against 'linear chain reporting routes' (1995: 67) where a victim only has access to a limited or single person to whom their concerns can be given. This can block the reporting of abuse and delay matters. Junior staff can feel equally powerless in reporting crimes to the police. Williams advocates a 'reporting web' (1995: 67) in which the individual with learning disabilities has access to a wide range of individuals, all of whom feel confident that it is their responsibility to report suspicions or allegations.

At a broader level of prevention, the voices of people with learning disabilities are going 'public' with drama performances given to audiences live or on video. The drama group, Change, composed of London-based members with learning disabilities, has put in dramatic form the 'case' of an abused woman, the police response and court processes.

Bearder and Ball (1997) employ dance and drama in a preventive but also empowering way, building on the points made at a conference of service users addressing the development of policies and guidelines on abuse. This work involves people with severe learning disabilities who attend a day centre; the dramatic performance emphasises the fundamental message that is to 'tell' if you are being abused or hurt. In a useful piece of evaluation the researchers found that people with learning disabilities had 'picked up' the key point of the performance about the importance of telling a 'boss' or manager and they suggest that its impact stemmed from the visual, accessible and creative medium employed of a combination of dance and drama. This format allows the voices of people with learning disabilities to be engaged in the debate about protection rather than having professionals reinforce their vulnerabilities. Strategies of avoiding dangers or preventing matters escalating can be learned through such approaches.

People with profound and complex disabilities, together with communication difficulties, are more likely to be victims of sexual abuse than other individuals (Campbell *et al.* 1996), though if and how sexual abuse is associated with other forms of abuse is not yet clear. As Campbell *et al.* acknowledge there may exist staff subcultures that on the 'lighter side' can be interpreted as joking, name calling or initiation rites (1996: 90). Residents, however, may perceive these as confusing, humiliating or terrifying. Listening to individuals when they are given time to talk together about general experiences within an institutional setting may be an important means of uncovering such distress; while inspectors can exercise this function it is also a role for those commissioning the service as care managers or health purchasers.

Supporting survivors

A small number of accounts now exist outlining the possible support available to people who have been abused. Some focus on support through the process of disclosure, investigation and prosecution. Bonniface (the founder of Voice) and Fraser (1994), for example, report the lessons learned from the support of a young woman who survived sexual abuse in a residential home. Bonniface, the survivor's mother, also reveals her own need for help – practically and emotionally – to survive the experience of learning of her daughter's pain and the trauma enforced by the experience.

Bonniface and Fraser (1994) identify that 'Nicky' (the young woman) initially blamed herself for the assault 'saying "I wasn't naughty, was I?"' (1994: 97). She seemed to talk to her abuser in a threatening way. Her mother thought that she both wanted to be believed and the abuser to be punished (1994: 98):

> When the verdict was announced, the look on my daughter's face of sheer delight was indeed a joy to behold. She had not been present in court after the first day so, on seeing the verdict on television, she jumped up and clapped, saying that she was right and that he was not going to hurt her now, was he?
>
> (1994: 101)

This example shows the impact of a resolution to the experience of abuse and demonstrates the need for both the victim of the crime and family members for support to develop and identify their self-perception as survivors.

Speaking out in court

The difficulties of the court-room experience itself have been well documented by Voice. Many of these centre on the adversarial contest and opaque legal language, bearing similarities to critiques developed by other victim interest groups. Piecemeal reforms, such as the possibility of the siting of screens between defendant and witness have been recently introduced. New support services, including the opportunity to visit the court prior to the trial, are at times available. Voice's (Hollins *et al.* 1994) booklet, *Going to Court*, tells the story of a witness in pictures and takes readers through the process of the report of an incident to the trial hearing. Using the perspective of the complainant with learning disabilities, this guide conveys a sense of the fear and uncertainty of the court appearance and also illustrates the delays possible.

The need for personal support as well as information is frequently identified. This may be available from generic organisations who provide services to members of the public, such as Victim Support schemes or Witness Support schemes, based in Crown Courts. Cohen (1998) reports a variety of good local practice with liaison between a Witness Support Service and court officials to make them aware of a witness's special needs, notably the need for simple and appropriate phrasing and questioning. The experience of the individual with learning disabilities and the impact and meaning of the court environment and its process is often seen to be negative; the counterbalance to this is generally to try to make personal connections to increase familiarity, to provide a link-person or guide and to explain the process step by step.

One particular reform that has been urged is extension of the right available to children to give evidence by video link. The Director of Public Prosecutions, Dame Barbara Mills (1998), drew attention to another facet of video recording: its use to convince the Crown Prosecution Service (CPS) that a case offered a realistic prospect of conviction. She advised close and early co-operation with the police and gave, by example, the case of a woman who had been assaulted in a day centre by a member of staff. Here, the police had interviewed her on videotape for the benefit of the Crown Prosecution Service, the organisation making the decision about prosecutions. This video was not for court use but had been shown to the CPS to demonstrate the complainant's abilities when well-prepared and also her determination. In such ways individuals' experiences can be used constructively to promote justice and a sense of security, as well as increasing the likelihood of securing a conviction and so protecting others.

Establishing a voice

Prominent in discussions about the abuse of people with learning disabilities in the UK is Voice, a pressure group that describes itself as 'a support and action group for people with learning disabilities who have been abused aimed at supporting families and gaining awareness' (Voice 1997). Voice is a membership organisation, largely composed of parents whose adult son or daughter has been sexually abused. In terms of its support to such parents it offers a self-help function, with personal contact and a newsletter. The newsletter describes the rationale for the development of parent contact points:

> We felt that parents might find it helpful to talk to other parents who had themselves suffered the trauma of abuse. ... All the parents felt strongly that they wanted to help. Their own son or daughter had been abused and their whole family had suffered and while this had happened and could never be altered they wanted to try to prevent other individuals and families suffering the same pain and trauma in the future.
>
> (1997: 5)

Voice has been particularly successful in operating in the political arena with its development of an All Party Parliamentary Support Group, which offers a means of promoting the issue of abuse on the political agenda and developing influential contacts and channels of communication.

It is possible to see Voice as successful at a number of levels: it has certainly provided many parents or relatives with a credible and, by their own accounts, supportive grouping. Operating at a political level, it promotes opportunities for relatives' accounts to reach the ears of policy-makers. The level of experience among its parent members is high and the organisation can argue its points with credibility. Voice's Director, Christina Horrocks (1998), for example, conveys the message from parents that criminal prosecution is a positive response (as appropriate) and that Voice members support prosecution despite the 'legal hurdle race'. The power of such stories of abuse as collected by Voice describes graphically the pain, trauma, anxiety, guilt and disbelief of parents whose children have been victimised. One father wrote:

> Someone has violated a part of me and I feel a deep, deep anger mixed with dreadful fears for her future and a sense of gross injustice that wants to shout from my very soul, and to open people's eyes to the real truth, not the truth of convenience, the one that safeguards their interests, but the truth of decency that understands the confused and frightened feelings of a young girl who was not in a position of judging or even comprehending the wrong that has been perpetrated on herself.
>
> (1998: 20)

It is important, though, to begin to differentiate between the views of people with learning disabilities and those of their families or carers. Such distinctions have featured strongly in discussions about care and risk-taking rather more than direct discussions about abuse. As noted earlier, relatives have often acted to bring abuse to public attention and they have expressed their feelings and drawn attention to the emotional and physical harm perpetrated on their relatives.

In the UK, so far the most articulate relatives of victims of abuse have been their parents, confirming their pre-eminence as carers for those living in the community but also their role as parents when their adult child has left home to live in residential care. While there may be no legal framework for their role, the norms of family responsibility appear heightened in such circumstances and, while no official guardianship status exists, it is clear that many parents see themselves as interested and involved in decisions about care and its quality. Many of them, for example, will have been involved in the choice of residential provision and may be contributing financially to the home. The account presented by Fitton *et al.* (1995), describing how two young women with profound and multiple disabilities achieved a home of their own, provides an illustration of the role of parents in setting out to establish a home for their daughters that provided good-quality care and a high degree of empowerment. In this example very clear lines of communication and procedures were set up to reduce the possibility of abuse.

Not all experience is so positive and much negative feeling may arise from carers' different perspectives on risk-taking and the imperatives of residential life. Carers in particular have been critical of the quality of residential care provided on a long- or short-term basis. As Nolan *et al.* (1996) observe, many carers hold a strong belief that they alone can provide good-quality, individualised care. Some avoid talking about the subject and residential care becomes a 'taboo' subject (1996: 127). In 'constructing' the identity of their adult child as one that focuses on abilities, positive characteristics and human dignity, carers of adult children with learning disabilities can feel cruelly let down by services that neglect the individuality they have tried hard to maintain and develop. Hubert's study of respite care illustrates some of these feelings. One mother described her distress at the service provided: 'Each time he comes home with little things wrong, and they're minor things to other people ... but it just aggravates me and I feel I'm doing him down by sending him back there' (1991: 40).

Other tensions may arise when carers do not share the residential home's policy on positive risk-taking. Heyman *et al.* (1998), for example, explore how many parents see venturing outside as 'risky'; staff, however, view such attitudes as over-protective and stifling. Staff are optimistic that service users will learn from mistakes; parents see themselves picking up the pieces if harm occurs.

Such differences in perspective may form an undercurrent of discussions but a unifying perspective has been discernible where debate has focused on extreme examples of abuse. The growing articulation of service users and users of residential services with learning disabilities may challenge this consensus. A study of self-advocacy (Mitchell 1997), for example, points to the difficulties experienced by people with learning disabilities in being perceived as adults. Individuals reported that they had restrictions placed on them by their parents and that they had little control or independence. It may be that residential care can be liberating to some extent and a focus on its potential to be abusive may not sit with individual experiences of alternatives.

Users' perspectives on residential services remain under-articulated and their increasing involvement in quality assurance mechanisms and inspection looks set to offer much in teaching non-users what is important and meaningful. Users' and carers' views may differ, of course, and this is now generally anticipated as a possibility. Much less is known though of differences between users and how they may hold different understandings of residential life. Their views and experiences need to be brought centre-stage both to highlight abusive environments but also to challenge what constitutes abuse.

References

Atkinson, D. (1988) 'Mentally handicapped', in I. Sinclair (ed.) *Residential Care: The Research Reviewed*, London: National Institute for Social Work.
—— (1994) 'Group-based reminiscence with people with learning difficulties', in J. Bornat (ed.) *Reminiscence Reviewed: Perspectives, Evaluations and Achievements*, Buckingham: Open University Press.
Azmi, S., Emerson, E., Caine, A. and Hatton, C. (1996) *Improving Services for Asian People with Learning Disabilities and their Families*, Manchester: Hester Adrian Research Centre.
Barron, D. (1987) 'Locked away', *Community Living* 1(2): 8–9.
Bearder, C. and Ball, L. (1997) 'Towards educating adults with learning disabilities on issues of abuse: A report of an innovative use of dance, drama and mime', *Journal of Learning Disabilities* 1(3): 120–30.
Bewley, C. (1997) *Money Matters: Helping People with Learning Difficulties Have More Control Over Their Money*, London: Values into Action.
Bonniface, J. and Fraser, G. (1994) 'Supporting a survivor: Lessons to be learned', in J. Harris and A. Craft (eds) *People with Learning Disabilities at Risk of Physical or Sexual Abuse*, Kidderminster: British Institute of Learning Disabilities.
Booth, T., Simons, K. and Booth, W. (1990) *Outward Bound: Relocation and Community Care for People with Learning Difficulties*, Buckingham: Open University Press.
Buckinghamshire County Council (1998) *Independent Longcare Inquiry*, Buckingham: Buckinghamshire County Council.
Cambridge, P. (1998) 'The physical abuse of people with learning disabilities and challenging behaviours: Lessons for commissioners and providers', *Tizard Learning Disability Review* 3(1): 18–27.
Campbell, M., Cullen, C. and Parry, A. (1996) *Approaches to People with Profound and Complex Disabilities*, St Andrews, Scotland: University of St Andrews.
Cohen, P. (1998) 'Helping hands', *Community Care*, 12 February: 18–19.
Committee of Inquiry (1969) *Report of the Committee of Inquiry into Allegations of Ill-Treatment of Patients and other Irregularities at the Ely Hospital, Cardiff*, Cmd 3975, London: HMSO.
Committee of Inquiry into Farleigh Hospital (1971) *Report of the Committee of Inquiry into Farleigh Hospital*, London: HMSO.

Committee of Inquiry into Normansfield Hospital (1978) *Report of the Committee of Inquiry into Normansfield Hospital*, Cmd 7357, London: HMSO.

Committee of Inquiry into South Ockenden Hospital (1974) *Report of the Committee of Inquiry into South Ockenden Hospital*, London: HMSO.

Cooper, M. (1997) 'Mabel Cooper's life story', in D. Atkinson, M. Jackson and J. Walmsley (eds) *Forgotten Lives: Exploring the History of Learning Disability*, Kidderminster: British Institute of Learning Disability.

Corkish, C. and Heyman, B. (1998) 'The resettlement of people with severe learning difficulties', in B. Heyman (ed.) *Risk, Health and Health Care*, London: Arnold.

Fido, R. and Potts, M. (1997) 'Using oral histories', in D. Atkinson, M. Jackson and J. Walmsley (eds) *Forgotten Lives: Exploring the History of Learning Disability*, Kidderminster: British Institute of Learning Disabilities.

Fitton, P., O'Brien, C. and Willson, J. (1995) *Home at Last: How Two Young Women with Profound Intellectual and Multiple Disabilities Achieved Their Own Home*, London: Jessica Kingsley.

Heyman, B., Huckle, S. and Handyside, E. (1998) 'Freedom of the locality for people with learning difficulties', in B. Heyman (ed.) *Risk Health and Health Care*, London: Arnold.

Hollins, S., Sinason, V. and Bonniface, J. (1994) *Going to Court*, Derby: Voice.

Horrocks, C. (1998) 'What's happening in practice? The perspectives of victims and families', paper presented at 'Fair Hearing: Justice for People with Learning Difficulties' Conference, 12 February, London.

Hubert, J. (1991) *Home Bound: Crisis in the Care of Young People with Severe Learning Disabilities*, London: King's Fund Centre.

Law Commission (1995) *Mental Incapacity*, London: HMSO, Law Com No. 231.

Malin, N. (1997) 'Policy to practice: A discussion of tension, dilemma and paradox in community care', *Journal of Learning Disabilities for Nursing, Health and Social Care* 1(3): 131–40.

Martin, J. (1984) *Hospitals in Trouble*, Oxford: Blackwell.

Mental Health Foundation (1996) *Building Expectations: Opportunities and Services for People with a Learning Disability*, London: Mental Health Foundation.

Millard, L. (1994) 'Between ourselves: Experiences of a women's group on sexuality and sexual abuse', in A. Craft (ed.) *Practice Issues in Sexuality and Learning Disabilities*, London: Routledge.

Mills, B. (1998) 'The role of the Crown Prosecution Service', paper presented at 'Fair Hearing: Justice for People with Learning Difficulties' Conference, 12 February, London.

Mitchell, P. (1997) 'The impact of self-advocacy on families', *Disability and Society* 12(1): 43–56.

Nolan, M., Grant, G. and Keady, J. (1995) *Understanding Family Care*, Buckingham: Open University Press.

Potts, M. and Fido, R. (1991) *A Fit Person to be Removed: Personal Accounts of Life in a Mental Deficiency Institution*, Plymouth: Northcote House Publishers.

Ramcharan, P. (1998) *Residents' Rights for People with Learning Disabilities Living in Large Hospitals*, Bangor Centre for Social Policy Research and Development, University of Wales, Summer: 5–8.

Reynolds, L. (1989) 'My own perspective and experience', in A. Brechin and J. Walmsley (eds) *Making Connections*, London: Hodder & Stoughton.

Sinason, V. (1994) 'Working with sexually abused individuals who have a learning disability', in A. Craft (ed.) *Practice Issues in Sexuality and Learning Disabilities*, London: Routledge.

Voice (1997) *Voice UK Newsletter*, August.

—— (1998) 'A father's view from the heart', in *One Aim, One Voice – Guidance Booklet*, Derby: Voice.

Wagner Report (1988) *Residential Care: A Positive Choice*, London: HMSO.

Walmsley, J. (1997) 'Telling the history from local sources', in D. Atkinson, M. Jackson and J. Walmsley (eds) *Forgotten Lives: Exploring the History of Learning Disability*, Kidderminster: British Institute of Learning Disabilities.

Williams, C. (1995) *Invisible Victims: Crime and Abuse Against People with Learning Difficulties*, London: Jessica Kingsley.

6 The abuse of adults in mental health settings

Jennie Williams and Frank Keating

The safety of people using mental health services has often been assumed and even romanticised in the myth of the pastoral mental hospital (Stevenson and Carson 1995). This is no longer the case, and in this chapter we consider the abuse of adults in a range of psychiatric settings, including in-patient services, counselling and therapy. The central argument of this chapter is that abuse in psychiatric services is closely linked to the existence of social inequalities, and is best understood and addressed from a perspective that takes this into account. We draw upon knowledge from a range of sources, including our involvement with a national organisation addressing professional abuse and a study of abuse in two local authorities.

Defining the problem

Johnson (1986), cited in Sobsey (1994), argues that we need a common definitional frame of reference before we can build and evaluate knowledge in a particular field. More specifically, he suggests that it is only when we adopt a standard definition of abuse that a causal theory of abuse can be explored. We agree, but this is not easy to achieve in the context of mental health services, when many of the central functions are abusive. This has been discussed, for example, in relation to compulsory detention and treatment (e.g. Cohen 1994; Campbell 1998), to the use of medication to silence and ignore human distress (e.g. Breggin 1993) and to the widespread failure of services to acknowledge and respond to the needs of patients (e.g. Coleman 1998; Sassoon and Lindow 1995). Such concerns are well-grounded, and continue to energise the service user movement in the UK and other countries: 'I believe there is one commonality that does exist and that is the shared oppression that psychiatric practice inflicts on users' (Coleman 1998). Against this background, we propose the following definition of abuse that acknowledges that abuse can be situated in inequitable relations between individuals, and between groups. As such, it invites consideration of the broader social context: 'Abuse is the use of power to serve self-interest (or group interest) when there are seriously damaging consequences for a person (or group) that is less powerful.'

Perpetrators do not have to be aware of the damaging consequences of their actions for it to be abuse. Ideologies protect social groups that exploit and mistreat those who are less powerful (Williams and Watson 1988) and many individuals who behave abusively have self-protecting explanations and justifications for their behaviour. This latter point has been particularly well-documented by people working in the field of domestic violence (Gondolf 1998), but equally applies to perpetrators in the human services. For example, a common justification for sexual contact given by therapists is that sexual contact would help their clients (e.g. Benowitz 1994), or that there was mutual attraction and that clients are consenting adults (Gartrell and Sanderson 1994). Indeed, Simon and Epstein (1990) suggest that therapists who exploit thrive on self-deception.

As we note elsewhere (Williams and Watson 1988), power can have a range of bases. These include physical, financial, social status and position. These powers can be used in a range of ways to serve self (or group) interest at the expense of those using psychiatric services. POPAN (Prevention of Professional Abuse Network), the national organisation concerned with abuse by health and social care workers, uses the following empirically derived categories: sexual abuse, emotional abuse, physical abuse, racial abuse, financial abuse and institutional abuse. There is also evidence to support the addition of neglect (Potier 1993) and breaking confidentiality (Darley *et al.* 1994) to this list.

Understanding the silence

There has been long-standing recognition of the possibility of health care workers abusing their powers. The Hippocratic Oath, written over 2,000 years ago, and a variety of codes since then have all explicitly forbidden health care professionals and practitioners to exploit the power they have in relation to their patients. In the current context there are statutory duties on professionals to protect the interests of people with mental health problems. For example, it is an offence for any staff member to ill-treat or wilfully neglect an in-patient or out-patient (Section 127 (1) of the Mental Health Act, 1983). It is also an offence for any person who is charged with the care of a vulnerable adult to engage in sexual activity with them (Section 128 (1) of the 1959 Mental Health Act, which was not repealed).

However, this formal recognition of risk has not been accompanied by a proactive stance towards abuse in mental health services. Although service user complaints about psychiatric services within hospitals have a long history (Campbell 1996), the shift to community services has given this a new impetus. Much of this new interest and research focuses on therapy and counselling, and comparatively little attention has been directed to abuse within mainstream mental health services. To date there has been no study in the UK to establish the incidence and prevalence of abuse in mental health services. Furthermore, in a climate of increased concern about the abuse of vulnerable clients within human services, there are indications that mental health services are especially unwilling to address the issue. In a study to develop, implement, monitor and evaluate adult protection policies (Brown and Stein 1997; Brown and Keating 1998) we found that the levels of reporting abuse in mental health services were much lower in comparison to other client groups. There were indications that this was because mental health practitioners were particularly unlikely to report abuse. In a focus group that provided a multidisciplinary group of mental health practitioners with opportunities to comment in more depth on the issue, they offered a range of explanations for not officially recording incidents of abuse. These included: 'if we have to log abuse, we will be doing it all the time' (focus group participant).

The reluctance of staff to report incidents was also found by Crowner *et al.* (1994). In this study, video cameras were used to record incidents of violence in an intensive-care psychiatric unit. Over the period of assessment, 155 incidents of assault were recorded; however, only twelve incidents were reported. Some of the factors that contribute to the apparent reticence of mental health services to address issues of abuse will now be considered.

First, addressing issues of abuse in the context of psychiatry is particularly difficult. This is, we believe, because one of the prime functions of the institution is to rename and manage the psychological damage and distress caused by social inequalities. As a social institution, psychiatry, like other institutions, protects the interests of those who are already powerful and privileged in our society. The most important way in which it fulfils this function and helps preserve the social *status quo*, is by obscuring and denying the role of social inequalities in the aetiology and maintenance of mental health difficulties. This case is persuasively argued by writers such as Penfold and

Walker (1984) and Szasz (1961). It is also the most parsimonious explanation for the huge resistance within psychiatry to taking account of the convincing evidence documenting the impact of social inequalities, such as gender, 'race', class, sexuality and age on mental health, and on mental health provision. There is now a vast literature tracking the impact of social inequalities on mental health through poverty, sexual and physical abuse, and other profound experiences of powerlessness and loss (see Williams *et al.* 1993; Fernando 1995). However, this work rarely informs the thinking of people working within psychiatry. This means that staff have little support to understand how abuses of power bring people to mental health services. Instead, they are reliant on biochemical and intra-psychic models of distress, and labels such as 'schizophrenia', 'depression' and 'manipulative behaviour'. In short, much of the training, education and socialisation available to mental health workers undermines their capacity to identify and name behaviour as abusive, or to understand its roots in inequalities of power between individuals and social groups. This analysis helps to explain common difficulties associated with addressing abuse in psychiatric services and can help give direction to attempts to intervene and prevent abuse in these settings.

Second, like other client groups receiving human services, the low status and vulnerability of people using mental health services has been a factor in the lack of public interest shown in their welfare. Additionally, people with mental heath problems are usually portrayed as dangerous, aggressive individuals who need to be isolated to protect and safeguard the interests of society. There is little emphasis on the risk of harm by others to which service users may be exposed in institutions, community settings and the homes of people. Risk is associated with the 'mad' and the 'bad', and not within the institutions where they live and receive services. It is comparatively easy for the problem to be located in the least powerful partners in the psychiatric enterprise: patients and clients.

Third, when people using mental health services speak out about abuse, one of the difficulties they often have to contend with is that what they say is often not considered to be reliable and credible (Potier 1993; Lindow 1991; Williams and Lindley 1996). Instead, their observations, reports and complaints are attributed to their mental states. In the context of the inequality that exists between those who use and those who provide mental health services, this must be seen as an excuse rather than a reason for not taking action. There is now widespread recognition that people using mental health services are valid commentators on the quality of care, and logically this should include their experiences of, and opinions about, the safety of services.

Fourth, people involved in the provision of mental health services have to define behaviour as abusive, and we have already noted that this is difficult in a system that is finely tuned to ignoring issues relating to power and abuse. In addition, not only do they have to define behaviour as abusive, but also this knowledge needs to be shared and acted upon. A range of factors has been identified as affecting the capacity and inclination of staff to raise the alarm when they perceive a situation or an incident as abusive. This includes organisational variables such as overwork, low pay, staff burn-out and lack of safeguards for staff who are whistle-blowers. In addition, staff may not report abuse due to fear of reprisal from senior staff, loss of professional relationships, fear of 'losing face' should allegations be unfounded or being perceived as a troublemaker (Garrett 1998). Finally, people working within mental health services can feel overwhelmed by the scale of the problem, and feel powerless, disaffected and cynical (Ussher 1991; Williams and Lindley 1996).

Reaction

With the exceptions of official inquiries such as those into Ashworth Hospital (Blom-Cooper 1992), and the death of Orville Blackwood (Prins *et al.* 1993), the impetus to address the problem of abuse within mental health services has mainly come from outside statutory services. The emergence of an international mental health service user movement has been associated with service users speaking openly about their experiences of abuse in the mental health services. The most active response to this information has been from the independent and voluntary sector, where a range of organisations (e.g. MIND 1992; Southwark Community Health Council 1993; WISH (Women in Special Hospitals) 1993; POPAN 1998a) have become involved in directing attention to this problem and in action to improve the safety of mental health services. For example, abuse was identified as an important issue in the MIND 'Stress on Women' campaign in 1992, when over 30,000 leaflets called 'Your right to say No!' were distributed within psychiatric services (Darton *et al.* 1994). Since then there has been continuing media interest in the problem; the television campaigner Esther Rantzen did much to draw attention to the risk of sexual abuse within mental health services. Early on, women in local communities, Community Health Councils and other groups lobbied mental health services providers to develop a more effective response to sexual assault and abuse in services, and in some instances worked with them on the development of policies and guidance (Copperman and Burrowes 1992). POPAN, the national organisation concerned with abuse by health and social care workers, was established in 1992. Such efforts have been validated and informed by a growing international literature on abuse in therapy and counselling (for a review see Schoener *et al.* 1990); and the growing evidence that abuse is widespread in other services provided for vulnerable people (e.g. Crossmaker 1991; Morris 1993).

One issue that has attracted particular attention has been the risks to women living on the same wards and hospitals as violent men (Potier 1993; WISH 1993; Williams *et al.* 1998). Anxiety about risks to women has led to campaigns to prevent the integration of female and male wards, and to promote the development of women-only residential options (Wood and Copperman 1996). The relatively meagre published research on this specific issue (Hingley and Goodwin 1994) does suggest that women and men prefer to live separately and this is impacting on guidance (e.g. Department of Health 1996), even if it is slow to impact on service provision (Warner and Ford 1998).

The changes we have noted here indicate that there is a shift in consciousness about this issue and a growing willingness to take action. However, this impetus for change has largely come from outside mental health services, from groups representing the interests of mental health service users, women, and survivors of therapist abuse. Mental health services are not leading the way in directing attention to abuse, or in taking the safety of patients seriously.

Prevalence

Though the research base concerned with abuse in mental health services is still quite modest, it consistently confirms the seriousness of the problem. An early American study (Nibert *et al.* 1989) reported that 71 per cent of patients had been threatened with violence whilst inside a psychiatric institution. Fifty-three per cent reported that they had been physically assaulted and 38 per cent reported that they had been sexually assaulted inside a psychiatric institution.

A two-year action research project (Brown and Stein 1997), in which one of the authors (FK) was involved, offers further insights into the problem of abuse in mental health services. This project was funded by the Nuffield Foundation and focused on the development and implementation of adult protection policies in two local authorities in the UK. Professionals across a range of services were requested to document reported incidents of abuse in their agencies. Participants working within mental health services raised particular concerns around issues of definition, incidents of prior abuse, thresholds for abuse, reporting structures and confidentiality (Brown and Keating 1998). Key research questions for this study were: are the policies reaching all client groups, all types of abuse and all types of settings; what patterns of mistreatment are reported and what responses are documented? Mental health cases accounted for 14 per cent of the total number of reported cases ($N = 396$). Multiple abuse ranked the highest, which indicates that different types of abuse often co-occur. Staff were listed as the alleged perpetrator of the abuse in a high proportion of cases (30 per cent). The study found that most of the cases were already known to services. This raises concerns for those individuals who are not in contact with services and the structures or systems that are needed to make it possible for them to report incidents of abuse. This study also found different reasons for abuse in home settings compared to abuse in formal care settings. Abuse in home settings was found to be associated with poor-quality relationships, a carer's inability to provide care and outside pressures such as finances, findings similar to those noted by Penhale and Kingston (1997). Abuse in formal care was found to take place due to inadequately trained staff, poor supervision of staff, use of rigid or routine practices and staff workloads, findings similar to those reported by Williams (1995).

In 1996 the Mental Health Act Commission in collaboration with the Sainsbury Centre for Mental Health carried out a one-day visit of almost half ($N = 309$; 47 per cent) of the acute psychiatric wards in England and Wales (see Warner and Ford 1998). Particular attention was given to collecting data about the safety of women. The findings of the survey are depressing, but are unlikely to be surprising to anyone who has first-hand knowledge of these types of services. There was little indication that campaigns against mixed-sex wards were having an impact: 94 per cent ($N = 291$) of the units surveyed were found to be of this type. Seventy-three per cent of these wards had some procedures and practices in place that addressed the safety needs of women. However, this did not constitute an adequate response to the problem, as 57 per cent of staff reported that women patients were sexually harassed. Sexual harassment included disinhibited behaviour and remarks, exploitation of vulnerable women, verbal harassment, watching or following women, exposing/nudity of male patients and sexual assault.

Abuse by therapists, as Bouhoutsos (1984) notes, has been a source of public as well as private concern in North America since the 1970s, and this is evident in the extensive literature on the subject. Key findings are that between 5 and 10 per cent of psychiatrists, psychologists and social workers are prepared to acknowledge sexual contact with clients (e.g. Szymanska and Palmer 1993); that the incidence for male therapists is consistently much higher than that for women therapists (e.g. Schoener *et al.* 1990); that over 90 per cent of those abused by health care workers are women (Bouhoutsos 1984: 209); and that substantial numbers (ranging from 37 per cent to 80 per cent) of therapists who abuse are serial abusers (Bouhoutsos *et al.* 1983). In Britain abuse of clients by health and social care workers and therapists is only just beginning to be documented. However, emerging findings are similar to those found in North America, including that at least 4 per cent of clinical psychologists report sexual contact with a client; that perpetrators are predominantly male and their victims female; and that the majority of practitioners who misuse their power in relation to clients do so more than once (POPAN 1998a). Evidence from both North American and UK research suggests that the risk of abuse and exploitation is not confined to any particular group of care workers or type of situation (Pope *et al.* 1993; POPAN 1998a).

Vulnerable individuals

Available evidence suggests that those people who are disadvantaged, mistreated and discriminated against within the wider society are also at risk within mental health services. The indifference shown by mental health services to the impact of social injustice on patients' lives and mental health, means that it is much more likely that social inequalities will be replicated than challenged within these services.

To illustrate, there is a growing body of evidence to suggest that people from Black and minority ethnic groups are especially vulnerable in psychiatric services. Browne (1995) carried out a study to explore perceptions about 'race' in two hospitals and found that 75 per cent of staff perceived Black patients as more likely to be dangerous. He examined case records in these institutions and found more common use of restraint among Black patients and higher levels of medication than for their White counterparts. This was a small-scale study and points to the need for further exploration of issues around inappropriate levels of medications and lack of guidelines on restraint. There is also evidence that mental health services are especially unsafe for lesbian and gay people (Brown 1996; Jackson 1998), and older people. Being a member of a disadvantaged social group or groups appears to be associated with the increased probability of receiving physical treatments, and a reduced probability of receiving effective psycho-social care.

Prior victimisation is also a risk factor for involvement with mental health services. Reviews of the research in this field (e.g. Williams *et al.* 1993; Goodman *et al.* 1997) indicate that many women using mainstream mental health services have histories of victimisation. Surveys find that between 34 and 51 per cent of respondents report histories of child physical abuse; between 20 and 54 per cent report histories of child sexual abuse; between 54 and 64 per cent report being physically abused as an adult; and between 21 per cent and 38 per cent report being sexually assaulted as an adult. Such histories are normative experiences in the lives of women who are living in high-security psychiatric services (Potier 1993; Adshead 1994; Warner 1996). Although the victimisation of women by men is the most common form of abuse, men also offend against boys and men (Draucker 1992), and abuse perpetrated by women is known to occur. To date, there has been less pressure for research into the mental health implications of the victimisation of men. Women and men with histories and experiences of victimisation are especially vulnerable when using mental health services. Many will find that their experience of victimisation is ignored. For example, one study (Rose *et al.* 1991) found that many patients when asked why they did not report incidents of abuse, said that they never told anyone about it because they had not been asked. Today, more mental health workers are likely to be aware that there are links between victimisation and mental distress. However, few have been trained to use this information in the interests of patients or clients. It is unsurprising, therefore, that there are increasing reports of staff responding to patients in ways that are considered to be abusive. This includes reports of minimising the significance of sexual abuse (e.g. Webster 1991) and using it as a label and as an explanation, rather than as a starting point for offering help (Warner 1996). The risks of abuse survivors receiving poor or abusive responses from psychiatry is considerable given the part the institution plays in obscuring the psychological distress associated with structural inequalities in our societies.

A prior history of sexual abuse has also been identified as a risk factor for sexual re-victimisation by other service users (Gutheil 1991) and staff. Eighty per cent of people reporting abuse by health and social workers to POPAN between 1997–8 had histories of childhood sexual abuse (POPAN 1998a).

Unsafe services

Berland and Guskin (1994) in a survey of a range of US psychiatric facilities found that more allegations were made against public hospitals, compared to private and community hospitals, as well as more instances of multiple allegations. Though there are obvious problems in using complaints as a reliable indicator of actual abuse, the existence of corroborative evidence does suggest that life in in-patient statutory services is particularly unsafe. UK forensic mental health services have a reputation for being especially unsafe places for women (Potier 1993; Warner 1996; Williams *et al.* 1998). In these settings, women live in close proximity to men who may be known perpetrators of sexual and other serious offences. Women are in the minority and often have an especially low status in these services; lodging a complaint within this setting is both difficult and unlikely to bring satisfaction. Some of these risks were highlighted in a recent review we carried out of a small low-security psychiatric unit (Williams *et al.* 1998). All the respondents with first-hand information about the unit expressed concern over the safety of women residents. Some respondents also expressed concern over the vulnerability of several male residents to sexual harassment and assault. These are some of the comments made by the staff and residents we interviewed:

> A few blokes are sex maniacs – at one point men were doing things to each other – tried it on with me once when I was a bit low. It's OK for men, but hard for women. One girl who's brain-damaged – all the men grab hold of her because she is helpless. She is checked by staff to prevent rape. She isn't right for this place.

> It (sex) is not consensual all the time. I don't know of rape, but patients are pressured into it.

> Women have sex for a cigarette, sometimes people take advantage.

> There is a double standard, staff are more sensitive to the sexual abuse of women patients.

> Some of the female nurses were concerned that male patients who had a history of sexual offences should not be on the ward with female patients. But I don't see this as a major problem.

The sexual aspect is the most worrying, particularly the issue of informed consent. We don't have adequate strategies.

(Williams *et al.* 1998: 10)

Given the serious implications of these observations, it was encouraging that there was commitment within this service to take action, and that the feasibility of developing a women-only service was under consideration.

Damaging consequences of abuse

Crossmaker (1991) makes the point that the effects of institutional abuse, and forced or coerced treatment in other mental health settings, are often similar to the effects of sexual abuse. This includes feelings of alienation, dependency and powerlessness. Evidence suggests that abuse in mental health services, including therapy and counselling, has serious consequences for most, if not all, of those who are abused. In relation to abuse by mental health practitioners one follow-up study (Bouhoutsos *et al.* 1983) in the US found that 90 per cent of people had been harmed, and this is confirmed by information gathered from those people who contact POPAN (POPAN 1998a). Adverse emotional consequences include feelings of vulnerability, worthlessness and distrust. In the longer term this type of abuse has been identified as the primary factor in unemployment, family break-up, drug and alcohol abuse. In the process of struggling to cope with these experiences, people can find themselves labelled 'manipulative', 'promiscuous', 'hard to place', 'evil', 'personality disordered'. Many people feel responsible for the abuse, and believe that they are at fault. Most people experience difficulties in speaking about their abuse, and those that speak out face the very real possibility that their reports will be disregarded, disbelieved or trivialised. People who have been abused by mental health workers are usually very distrustful of these services in future. As a result, they may not avail themselves of relevant sources of help, or if they do, they may be very challenging to service providers (DeLozier 1994).

Seeking redress

It is not easy for people using mental health services to complain about abuse, or to have their complaints taken seriously. They are typically in a powerless position in relation to service providers, and may well be dealing with a service that is functionally insensitive to anything to do with abuses of power (see Crossmaker 1991). There is evidence that staff refuse to listen to or believe reports of abuse on the grounds that they are symptoms of madness and/or attention seeking (see Potier 1993; Williams *et al.* 1998). Alternatively, they may believe an incident took place, but that the patient was somehow responsible, that it was 'consensual', 'provoked' or that 'they were asking for it'.

Lodging complaints of abuse against service providers is especially difficult. These are some of the experiences of people using POPAN, as recounted by one of the workers:

> She went to see the doctor who had referred her to this psychiatrist. The doctor was severe with her and told her that she was herself entirely to blame for the sexual activity. He said that she was a responsible adult, and that if she was to make any complaint against Dr X she could be sued for libel and as the court would only have her word for what took place, she would possibly be liable for a sum such as £100,000. She was, he said, lashing out at Dr X with these allegations because of some crisis in her present life.
>
> The solicitor and client now are taking a case through the courts. Legal aid has been granted; the client has had a gruelling intensive psychiatric assessment for damages; she has had to write a very difficult account of what happened. This has all been very shocking to her and traumatic and bringing up a lot of big feelings and fear and isolation.
>
> (Williams, J. 1995: 3)

Most survivors of abuse by health and social care workers do not pursue complaints or take legal action. Only 13 per cent (15) of the people who brought their cases to the attention of POPAN in 1997–8 had sought, or were seeking, redress through the courts (POPAN 1998b). One of the reasons suggested for this is that by the time someone feels sufficiently robust to cope with the draining and adversarial process of bringing a complaint they are then 'out of time'. Currently the law requires that a negligence action is brought within three years from the date when the cause of action accrued or 'the date of knowledge', that is, when the plaintiff becomes aware of the negligence. This limitation period works against the interests of people who have been abused in mental health services, who may need time both to name behaviour as 'abusive' and to gather the personal, informational and other resources necessary to bring a complaint. It should be noted that this limitation period does not apply to criminal charges, and that in some circumstances a petition can be made for it to be waived. These circumstances could include the mental state of the petitioner.

Intervening

One consequence of the reluctance of mental health services to address issues of abuse is that these services are well-placed to learn from developments that have been taking place elsewhere in the human services. For example, there is now considerable experience in responding to abuse within children's services (see Christine Barter's chapter in this volume) and services for people with learning disabilities (see Hilary Brown's chapter). In drawing upon these interventions, it is important that they are not only relevant but compatible with the social inequalities perspective that, we have argued here, is central to understanding and addressing abuse in psychiatry. This perspective does alert us to the potential problems of importing the 'protection' orientation into mental health. While there are issues of protection in situations when service users are extremely vulnerable, this approach leaves power relations unexamined and is not an effective response to people who feel alienated, dependent and powerless. In contrast, an empowerment approach, one grounded in good evidence about the ways in which an individual or group has been disempowered, encourages us to think creatively about what needs to happen for clients and staff to be empowered.

Naming the problem

The relationship between those who use and those who provide mental health services is one of inequality. One consequence of this inequality for service users is that reporting abuse can be risky and unrewarding (see Jeanette Copperman and Julie McNamara's chapter). There is ample evidence of complaints made by service users being disregarded or handled in ways that were ineffective, and which left them feeling punished and diminished. Effective interventions are those that empower service users. These could include the provision of independent advocacy and of safe opportunities for service users to share experiences together in the context of user groups and fora. While service users may need support to name abuse and to feel able to bring a complaint, they also need access to a fair system for making a complaint, and they need to know how to use this system. One way for mental health services to identify points for improvement in this realm is to review their complaints system jointly with service users. For

example, many service users may be unaware that a complaints proce-
dure exists, or it may be difficult to use. Currently the indications are
that mental health service users find the process of making a
complaint very difficult.

Evidence cited earlier indicates that interventions also need to target
staff, who are reluctant to report incidents of abuse. One approach is
to ensure, through training and involvement in policy development,
that staff feel able to take constructive action about abuse in services.
The effectiveness of these interventions will be to a large extent contin-
gent on their rewards and costs. It is important that staff feel that
action against abuse is supported by the service culture and the wider
organisation. In parts of Canada and the US, one response to the
failure to report has been to introduce mandatory reporting (Gallop
1998). The introduction of this legislation is said to be associated with
worries about what is reportable and about the personal consequences
of whistle-blowing.

Policies

There is evidence that policies can go some way to address abuse, but a
professional culture that does not take account of the disastrous
personal effects of abuse cannot be changed through policy development alone. It requires a service to link abuse with the inequalities and
injustices that people with mental health problems experience. Policies
can bring agreed understandings and common procedures; they help
to institute co-ordinating mechanisms and assist in identifying the
characteristics and parameters of abuse and abusive practice (Brown
and Cambridge 1997). Policies unfortunately cannot legislate for
contexts that are abusive by their very nature, and do not constitute an
effective response to institutional abuse. For example, there is little to
suggest that policies or changes in management are the solution to the
abusive culture of the Special Hospitals. Discussions about the way
forward now include the option of the reconfiguration of secure
forensic services.

Policies may be underpinned by good intentions, but there is a
danger that they may be paternalistic in their approach towards service
users. Protection policies may position service users as dependent individuals who need intervention by an external body. There are
situations where policies may be required to safeguard the interests of
extremely vulnerable individuals, but we would argue that the most
effective response to abuse is one that enables service users to take

control of the situation and make decisions in accordance with their competence.

Responding to the perpetrator

At the moment, professional bodies can withdraw registration from those found to behave abusively to clients, but this does not prevent them from practising. In a recent case (British Psychological Society Disciplinary Board 1998), a psychologist found guilty of professional misconduct with several patients was allowed voluntarily to withdraw his name from the Register of Chartered Psychologists, whilst retaining his membership and fellowship of the Society. This outcome was widely and critically reported in the press. The rationale for the decision was that it was easier to monitor the man's behaviour whilst he was a member of the Society. Whatever the wisdom of this reasoning, it does make it clear that there are only limited mechanisms available for controlling mental health professionals and practitioners who behave abusively. One response to this problem has been to call for compulsory registration of all those engaged in talking treatment so that those who abuse their power can be struck off and prevented from practising (Wood 1993).

Mental health services also have responsibilities for working with perpetrators whose abusive behaviour is associated with, or caused by, psychological difficulties. There is a developing literature in this field, which includes interventions with men who physically and sexually abuse family members (Miller and Bell 1996; Shamai 1996; Gondolf 1998), and with therapists and other mental health practitioners. As yet, few professional bodies offer guidelines or procedures to address the rehabilitation of perpetrators, yet this is an area in which service providers are likely to need help (Whitehead and Unger 1991).

Prevention

Equality within mental health services

There is little to suggest that the inequality of power that characterises relations between those who use and those who provide mental health services is associated with good outcomes for service users. Arguably, this situation has also not been in the interests of those who provide mental health services, the overwhelming majority of whom want to make a useful contribution to the lives of others. Abuse in mental health services is perpetuated and hidden by the inequality of power between those who provide and those who use the services. Genuine attempts to shift power to clients and patients so that they are no longer passive recipients of care, and become active partners in their care and in the development of mental health services, need to be supported. Service commitment to equality, fairness and safety need to be evident, especially to those clients who are very dependent on services, who may also need advocacy and support to bring a complaint.

To date, mental health services have helped to hide and manage the psychological consequences of the social inequalities within our society. As long as they continue to fulfil this function it will be very difficult to provide safe and effective services to people in distress. It is time for a radical shift in the relations between mental health services, society and the Government. This requires mental health workers owning research on inequalities and mental health, and refusing to provide care based on aetiological models which ignore the effects of abuse, discrimination and disadvantage. This is a goal worth struggling for; it tackles the problem of institutional abuse, and supports the development of services that are effective and intolerant of abuses of personal power.

Training

Training can provide relevant knowledge and serve as an effective means of achieving good practice. This can include helping staff to become more self-aware of the beliefs and assumptions that can lead to the abuse of patients (Simon and Epstein 1990; Gallop 1998). Brown and Stein (1997) suggest that staff should be trained to assess the level of risk, the extent of the abuse, the impact of the abuse, the intention of the perpetrator and the legal implications. This type of targeted training needs to be part of a broader strategy to create safe and effective services by transforming the knowledge base of mental health services.

Priority needs to be given to shift the knowledge base of mental health services away from theories and practices that marginalise and trivialise the impact of social inequalities on the lives of services users, to those which support staff to behave ethically (Williams and Watson 1996). The important sources of this knowledge are easy to identify. First, there are people with first-hand experience of using mental health services, including those who have been abused in this context. Second, there is well-established and extensive research literature on social inequalities and mental health. Third, many mental health projects in the UK and elsewhere provide services shaped by principles of equality that address the damage caused by social inequalities. With few exceptions (Holland 1995; Watson *et al.* 1996; Watters 1996), these services are to be found at the margins of psychiatry, and are less constrained by psychiatric ideologies and dogma. Finally, everyone working within mental health services will have personal knowledge of power and powerlessness, and of the personal and social responses to abuses of power, including those that have relevance for mental health. This personal knowledge needs to be valued and used.

Using these resources and effecting this change in the knowledge base of mental health services will help to ensure that services are both safer and more effective. Achieving this change will need support from national training bodies and organisations, coupled with a strategic approach from services to ensure these changes are supported through training and supervision, and the broader organisational culture.

Conclusion

It has been argued here that abuse in mental health services needs to be situated in the context of social inequalities. The abuse of power is sustained and authorised by social inequalities and is necessary for their continuation. Social inequalities are pervasive and abuse occurs in all our social institutions, including the mental health services and the family. When services are considered within this framework it can be argued that mental health services are inherently problematic, because their function is often greatly at odds with the needs of people experiencing mental health difficulties.

References

Adshead, G. (1994) 'Damage: Trauma and violence in a sample of women referred to a forensic service', *Behavioral Sciences and the Law* 12(3): 235–49.

Barnes, M. (1996) 'Challenging the culture; representing the rights of women in special hospitals', in C. Hemingway (ed.) *Special Women? The Experience of Women in the Special Hospital System*, Aldershot: Avebury.

Benowitz, M. (1994) 'Comparing the experiences of women clients sexually exploited by female versus male psychotherapists', *Women and Therapy* (15)1: 69–83.

Berland, D.I. and Guskin, K. (1994) 'Patient allegations of sexual abuse against psychiatric hospital staff', *General Hospital Psychiatry* 16(5): 335–9.

Blom-Cooper, L. (1992) *Report of the Committee of Inquiry into Complaints about Ashworth Hospital*, London: HMSO.

Bouhoutsos, J.C. (1984) 'Sexual intimacy between psychotherapists and clients: Policy implications for the future', in L.E. Walker (ed.) *Women and Mental Health Policy*, London: Sage.

Bouhoutsos, J., Holroyd, J., Lerman, H., Forer, B. and Greenberg, M. (1983) 'Sexual intimacies between psychotherapists and patients', *Professional Psychology: Research and Practice* 14(2): 185–96.

Boyce, K. (1998) 'Asserting difference: Psychiatric care in black and white', in P. Barker and B. Davidson (eds) *Psychiatric Nursing: Ethical Strife*, London: Arnold.

Breggin, P.R. (1993) *Psychiatric Drugs: Hazards to the Brain*, New York: Springer.

British Psychological Society Disciplinary Board (1998) 'Notices from the Disciplinary Board', *The Psychologist* 11(11): 555.

Brown, H. and Cambridge, P. (1997) 'Policies and their coherent contribution to decision-making', in P. Cambridge and H. Brown (eds) *HIV and Learning Disability*, Kidderminster: British Institute of Learning Disability.

Brown, H. and Keating, F. (1998) ' "We're doing it already": Adult protection in mental health services', *Journal of Psychiatric and Mental Health Nursing* 5(4): 273–80.

Brown, H. and Stein, J. (1997) *Implementing Adult Protection Policies*, Milton Keynes: The Open University.

Brown, L.S. (1996) 'Preventing heterosexism and bias in psychotherapy and counselling', in E.D. Rothblum and L.A. Bond (eds) *Preventing Heterosexism and Homophobia*, London: Sage.

Browne, D. (1995) 'Sectioning: The black experience', in S. Fernando (ed.) *Mental Health in a Multi-ethnic Society: A Multi-disciplinary Handbook*, London: Routledge.

Campbell, P. (1996) 'The history of the user movement in the United Kingdom', in T. Heller, J. Reynolds, R. Gomm, R. Muston and S. Pattison (eds), *Mental Health Matters: A Reader*, Milton Keynes: Macmillan/The Open University.

—— (1998) 'Mentally healthy acts', *OpenMind* 94(10), November/December: 10.

Cohen, L.J. (1994) 'Psychiatric hospitalisation as an experience of trauma', *Archives of Psychiatric Nursing* 8(2): 78–81.

Coleman, R. (1998) *Politics of the Madhouse*, Runcorn: Handsell.

Copperman, J. and Burrowes, F. (1992) 'Reducing the risk of assault', *Nursing Times* 88(26): 64–5.

Crossmaker, M. (1991) 'Behind locked doors – institutional sexual abuse', *Sexuality and Disability* 9(3): 201–19.

Crowner, M.L., Peric, G., Stepcic, F. and Van, O.E. (1994) 'A comparison of video cameras and official incident reports in detecting inpatient assaults', *Hospital and Community Psychiatry* 45(11): 1144–5.

Darley, B., Griew, A., McLoughlin, K. and Williams, J. (1994) *How to Keep a Clinical Confidence: A Summary of Law and Guidance on Maintaining the Patient's Privacy*, London: HMSO.

Darton, K., Gorman, J. and Sayce, L. (1994) *Eve Fights Back: The Successes of MIND's Stress on Women Campaign*, London: MIND Publications.

DeLozier, P.P. (1994) 'Therapist sexual misconduct', *Women and Therapy* 15(1): 55–67.

Department of Health (1996) *NHS The Patient's Charter: Mental Health Services*, London: Department of Health.

Doyle, C. (1997) 'Protection studies: Challenging oppression and discrimination', *Social Work Education* 16(2): 8–19.

Draucker, C.B. (1992) *Counselling Survivors of Childhood Sexual Abuse*, London: Sage.

Fernando, S. (ed.) (1995) *Mental Health in a Multi-ethnic Society: A Multidisciplinary Handbook*, London: Routledge.

—— (1996) 'Training of mental health professionals: Confronting racism and taking account of culture', paper presented at 'Working Across Cultures' Conference, St George's Hospital, London.

Gallop, R. (1998) 'Abuse of power in the nurse-client relationship', *Nursing Standard* 12(37): 43–7.

Garrett, T. (1998) 'Sexual contact between patients and psychologists', *The Psychologist* 11(5): 227–30.

Gartrell, N.K. and Sanderson, B.E. (1994) 'Sexual abuse of women by women in psychotherapy: Counselling and advocacy', *Women and Therapy* 15(1): 39–54.

Gondolf, E.W. (1998) 'Identifying and assessing men who batter', in E.W. Gondolf (ed.) *Assessing Woman Battering in Mental Health Services*, London: Sage.

Goodman, L.A., Johnson, M., Dutton, M.A. and Harris, M. (1997) 'Prevalence and impact of sexual and physical abuse', in M. Harris and C.L. Landis (eds) *Sexual Abuse in the Lives of Women Diagnosed with Serious Mental Illness*, London: Harwood Academic.

Gutheil, T.G. (1991) 'Patients involved in sexual misconduct with therapists: Is a victim profile possible?', *Psychiatric Annals* 21(11): 661–7.

Hingley, S.M. and Goodwin, A.M. (1994) 'Living with the opposite sex: The views of long-stay psychiatric patients', *British Journal of Clinical Psychology* 33(2): 183–92.

Holland, S. (1995) 'Interaction in women's mental health and neighbourhood development', in S. Fernando (ed.) *Mental Health in a Multi-ethnic Society: A Multi-disciplinary Handbook*, London: Routledge.

Jackson, C. (1998) 'Mad to be gay', *Mental Health Care* 1(7): 222.

Jorgenson, L.M. (1995) 'Rehabilitating sexually exploitative therapists: A risk management perspective', *Psychiatric Annals* 25(2): 118–22.

Kirkwood, C. (1993) 'Women's experiences of emotional abuse', in C. Kirkwood (ed.) *Leaving Abusive Partners*, London: Sage.

Lindow, V. (1991) 'Experts, lies and stereotypes', *The Health Service Journal*, 29 August.

Llewelyn, S. (1993) 'The sexual abuse of clients by therapists', *Clinical Psychology Forum* 54 (April), 26–9.

Mental Health Act 1959, London: HMSO.

Mental Health Act 1983, London: HMSO.

Miller, J. and Bell, C. (1996) 'Mapping men's mental health', *Journal of Community and Applied Social Psychology* 6(5): 317–27.

MIND (1992) *Stress on Women: Policy Paper on Women and Mental Health*, London: MIND.

Morris, J. (1993) *Independent Lives: Community Care and Disabled People*, London: Macmillan.

Nibert, D., Cooper, S. and Crossmaker, M. (1989) 'Assaults against residents of a psychiatric institution: Residents' history of abuse', *Journal of Interpersonal Violence* 4(3): 342–9.

Penfold, P.S. and Walker, G.A. (1984) 'Psychiatric ideology and its functions', in P.S. Penfold and G.A. Walker (eds) *Women and the Psychiatric Paradox*, Milton Keynes: The Open University.

Penhale, B. and Kingston, P. (1997) 'Elder abuse, mental health and later life: Steps towards an understanding', *Aging and Mental Health* 1(4): 293–304.

POPAN (1998a) *POPAN: Prevention of Professional Abuse Network Annual Report*, London: POPAN.

—— (1998b) *First Bi-Annual Monitoring Report: April 1998 to October 1998*, London: POPAN.

Pope, K.S., Sonne, J.L. and Holroyd, J. (1993) 'Appendix C: Therapist-patient sexual involvement: A review of the research', in *Sexual Feelings in Psychotherapy: Explorations for Therapists and Therapists-in-Training*, Washington, DC: American Psychological Association.

Potier, M.A. (1993) 'Giving evidence: Women's lives in Ashworth Maximum Security Psychiatric Hospital', *Feminism and Psychology* 3(3): 335–47.

Prins, H., Backer-Holst, T., Francis, E. and Keitch, I. (1993) *Report of the Committee of Inquiry into the Death in Broadmoor Hospital of Orville Blackwood and a Review of the Deaths of Two Other Afro-Caribbean Patients: Big, Black and Dangerous*, London: HMSO.

Rose, S.M., Peabody, C.G. and Stratigeas, B. (1991) 'Undetected abuse among intensive case management clients', *Hospital and Community Psychiatry* 42(5): 499–503.

Rothblum, E.D. and Bond, L.A. (1996) *Preventing Heterosexism and Homophobia*, London: Sage.

Sassoon, M. and Lindow, M. (1995) 'Consulting and empowering black mental health system users', in S. Fernando (ed.) *Mental Health in a Multiethnic Society: A Multi-disciplinary Handbook*, London: Routledge.

Schoener, G.R., Milgrom, J.H., Gonsiorek, J.C., Luepker, E.T. and Conroe, R.M. (1990) *Psychotherapist Sexual Involvement with Clients: Intervention and Prevention*, Minneapolis, Minnesota: Minneapolis Walk-in Counselling Center.

Shamai, M. (1996) 'Couple therapy with battered women and abusive men: Does it have a future?', in J.L. Edleson and Z.C. Eisikovits (eds) *Future Interventions with Battered Women and their Families*, London: Sage.

Simon, R. and Epstein, R. (1990) 'The exploitation index: An early warning indicator of boundary violations in psychotherapy', *Bulletin of the Menninger Clinic* 54: 450–65.

Sobsey, D. (1994) *Violence and Abuse in the Lives of People with Disabilities*, London: Jessica Kingsley.

Southwark Community Health Council (1993) *Prevention and Response: Sexual Violence and Abuse in Hospital Wards*, London: Southwark CHC.

Stevenson, V. and Carson, J. (1995) 'The pastoral myth of the mental hospital: A personal account', *International Journal of Social Psychiatry* 41(2): 147–51.

Szasz, T. (1961) *The Myth of Mental Illness*, New York: Hoeber–Harper.

Szymanska, K. and Palmer, S. (1993) 'Therapist–client sexual contact', *Counselling Psychology Review* 8(4): 22–33.

Ussher, J.M. (1991) 'Clinical psychology and sexual equality: A contradiction in terms?', *Feminism and Psychology* 1(1): 63–8.

Warner, L. and Ford, R. (1998) 'Conditions for women in in-patient psychiatric units: The Mental Health Act Commission 1996 national visit', *Mental Health Care* 11(7): 225–8.

Warner, S. (1996) 'Visibly special? Women, child sexual abuse and special hospitals', in C. Hemingway (ed.) *Special Women? The Experience of Women in the Special Hospital System*, Aldershot: Avebury.

Watson, G., Scott, C. and Ragalsky, S. (1996) 'Refusing to be marginalised: Groupwork in mental health services for women survivors of childhood sexual abuse', *Journal of Community and Applied Social Psychology* 6(5): 341–54.

Watters, C. (1996) 'Inequalities in mental health: The Inner City Mental Health Project', *Journal of Community and Applied Social Psychology* 6(5): 383–94.

Webster, M. (1991) 'Emotional abuse in therapy', *Australian and New Zealand Journal of Family Therapy* 12(3): 137–45.

Whitehead, J. and Unger, L. (1991) 'Bringing the abusive employee back', *Journal of Mental Health Administration* 18(2): 143–7.

Williams, C. (1995) *Invisible Victims: Crime and Abuse Against People with Learning Difficulties*, London: Jessica Kingsley.

Williams, J. (1995) 'Complaints procedures: Learning from complaints made about therapists and counsellors', presented at the World Federation of Mental Health World Congress, Dublin.

Williams, J., Field, V. and Fernando, S. (1998) *Review of the Newbridge Unit*, Canterbury: Tizard Centre.

Williams, J. and Lindley, P. (1996) 'Working with mental health service users to change mental health services', *Journal of Community and Applied Social Psychology* 6(1): 1–14.

Williams, J. and Watson, G. (1988) 'Sexual inequality, family life and family therapy', in E. Street and W. Dryden (eds) *Family Therapy in Britain*, Milton Keynes: The Open University.

—— (1996) 'Mental health services that empower women', in T. Heller, J. Reynold, R. Gomm, R. Muston and S. Pattison (eds) *Mental Health Matters: A Reader*, London: Macmillan/The Open University.

Williams, J., Watson, G., Smith, H., Copperman, J. and Wood, D. (1993) *Purchasing Effective Mental Health Service for Women: A Framework for Action*, London: MIND publications/Tizard Centre, University of Kent at Canterbury.

Winship, G. (1998) 'Democracy in psychiatric settings; collectivism vs. individualism', in P. Barker and B. Davidson (eds) *Psychiatric Nursing: Ethical Strife*, London: Arnold.

WISH (Women in Special Hospitals) (1993) 'Integration: In Whose Interest?' Conference, held in London, March.

Wood, D. (1993) *The Power of Words: Uses and Abuses of Talking Treatments*, London: MIND.

Wood, D. and Copperman, J. (1996) 'Sexual harassment and assault in psychiatric services', in R. Perkins, Z. Nadirshaw, J. Copperman and C. Andrews (eds) *Women in Context: Good Practice in Mental Health Services for Women*, London: Good Practices in Mental Health.

7 Institutional abuse in mental health settings

Survivor perspectives

Jeanette Copperman and Julie McNamara

This chapter will explore survivor perspectives on abuse using accounts drawn from survivors themselves. It will particularly focus on women's accounts of abuse in the mental health system. Women have been chosen as they are both over-represented within the mental health system and have been shown to be at the blunt end of many psychiatric practices. These include experiencing higher rates of electroconvulsive therapy (ECT), higher hospital admissions and less specialist input (Williams *et al.* 1993).

Women's accounts also highlight some of the ways in which power relations in society as a whole are both mirrored and exaggerated within the mental health system. Women are not the only group who receive unequal treatment. The preponderance of young Black men taken in by the police under Section 136 of the Mental Health Act, 1983 (Bean *et al.* 1991) and the over-medication of Black men and women in the psychiatric system (MIND 1992) all testify to the unequal power relations that characterise the mental health system.

Abuse has been exposed within a wide range of mental health settings. The recently revived inquiry into Ashworth Hospital has exposed serious abuse of power and reawakened interest in Special Hospitals. The Ashworth inquiry described the regime in the hospital as 'infantalising, demeaning and anti-therapeutic for women' (Blom-Cooper 1992). Whilst abuse within relatively closed institutions such as Ashworth has been exposed, other inquiries have shown that abuse is more widespread. For example, the lack of safety in mental health settings, violence and sexual harassment have been the focus of investigation and campaigns. A recent unannounced visit to 309 acute psychiatric wards by the Mental Health Act Commission found that in just over half the wards, staff identified problems of sexual harassment of women patients by male patients (Sainsbury Centre 1997). One of the accounts included in this chapter highlights some everyday experiences on a ward.

The context

It is tempting to think that the move to community care and into smaller settings will solve problems of abuse. There has been overwhelming support for de-institutionalisation from users of mental health services despite underfunding and patchy provision (Rogers *et al.* 1993). Whilst it appears to be true that in more open institutions there are more checks and balances, the stigmatisation of mental health service users and fundamental imbalances of power present issues in all settings. For example, sexual abuse in counselling and psychotherapy has been shown to be widespread. In one US study 15 per cent of male therapists admitted to sexual contact with clients, and of those who had had sexual contact, 75–80 per cent did so with more than one client and 92 per cent of the reports related to a male therapist and a female client (Bouhoustos *et al.* 1983). In a national study in the UK 4 per cent of clinical psychologists admitted to sexual contact with clients (Garrett 1992). According to the Prevention of Professional Abuse Network (POPAN):

> Many people have told no one and there isn't even a close friend to come forward on their behalf. The dynamics are complex and complicated but there is often a great similarity to what we know happens with incest, family secrets, protection of the abuser, confusion, shame and guilt.
>
> (Edwardes and Fasal 1992)

A crucial backdrop to the accounts in this chapter is the activity of a diverse and flourishing user-led movement. This includes local and national mental health advocacy and self-help organisations, such as the UK Advocacy Network and the work of campaigning organisations such as Survivors Speak Out. User-led groups have tended to centre their demands on the right to a choice of treatment, better information and the right to be treated as a whole person (Faulkner 1996). They have highlighted the routine over-medication and dehumanising treatment often meted out to psychiatric patients.

Since the mid-1980s there have also been several waves of campaigning, by women in particular, which have highlighted the particular abuse of women within the psychiatric system and the ways in which women's needs have been neglected and ignored. For example,

MIND's Stress on Women campaign (Darton, Gorman and Sayce 1994) highlighted issues of choice and safety for women. It focused particularly on making sexual harassment and assault within hospital wards and other mental health settings visible. POPAN, which provides advocacy and support to people who have been abused by counsellors, therapists and other professionals, has highlighted abuse in individual counselling and therapy. It has been collecting accounts and assisting women in taking complaints forward. The national Women and Mental Health Network has drawn together accounts from individuals and groups.

Without the activity of all these organisations much abuse would have remained invisible and without a name. Some of the accounts in this chapter are drawn from the UK-based Women and Mental Health Network publications.

Survivor perspectives

Definitions

Users and survivors are not a homogeneous group, as Wallcraft and Read (1994) point out:

> We have already referred to service users, patients and clients. We could have used recipients or survivors of psychiatry, or even consumers or customers. There is no one generic term that can take account of the different relationships people have with mental health services – from voluntary attenders of a drop-in, to people held against their will in secure units.

For some, the term survivor is of crucial importance:

> Survivor is a term I embrace with pride because it speaks of hope beyond despair, an existence in spite of life's traumas and, often, in spite of treatment received within the mental health services.
>
> (McNamara 1996: 198)

There is no one term that is acceptable to everyone so in this chapter the terms survivors and users of mental health services will be used.

The nature of abuse

Horrific individual abuses such as rapes and violent assaults do occur. Both survivors and workers would agree that these constitute violations, but abuse within the psychiatric system is seen by many survivors as based in a continuum of unequal power relations in a system rooted in containment, control and fear rather than as an individual aberrant phenomenon.

> During the three years I spent in institutions I saw and experienced a lot of abuse. Some of it was violent, some of it was more subtle, but it was almost always present in one form or another like a polluted river running through our lives. We did the best we could to survive. Many of us did not.
>
> (Dundas 1995: 35)

The continuing lack of belief that is accorded to survivor accounts of abuse, whether this is sexual abuse, emotional abuse or coercive treatment, is striking. For example, the Ashworth inquiry was precipitated by a television documentary that presented evidence that patient abuse was a commonplace but hidden characteristic of life at Ashworth Hospital. It highlighted the fact that out of 600 complaints made by patients at Ashworth over a ten-year period, not one had been upheld (*Cutting Edge* 1991). Workers who take up allegations of abuse can also find themselves disbelieved and marginalised. Helen Leibling, a clinical psychologist at the hospital, won damages against Ashworth Hospital – her employers – for sex discrimination and constructive dismissal. She had tried to take forward several complaints about sexual assault on women patients and the ill treatment of women who had complained (*Liverpool Daily Post* 1997).

A framework for discussion

It is clear from the accounts of survivors that the impact of abuse on an individual has to be understood in the light of their past experiences and that abuse of any form is harmful. For example, Ruth Ingram has pulled together research suggesting that 10 per cent of all women are currently experiencing violence from a known man and that 25 per cent of women admitted for emergency psychiatric care are experiencing such violence (Ingram 1993). There is considerable evidence that use of mental health services is linked to past abuse:

At least 50 per cent of women who use community and hospital based mental health services have been sexually and/or physically abused as children and adults. There is also strong evidence that sexual and physical abuse is at the core of much that is diagnosed as severe mental illness and that abuse is strongly linked with high service use.

(Williams and Watson 1994)

Survivors have identified the ways in which forced treatment and dehumanising practices echo the abuse that brought them to mental health services in the first place. This will be the topic of the first section, which will explore the legal framework and the organisational culture that set up a situation where some practices which would be seen as abusive in any other setting become 'normal' in mental health institutions.

Sexual abuse and safety within mental health services are explored in the second section. We include part of an account of a sexual assault in a hospital by a staff member and the institution's subsequent response to it. An extract from 'Turning Tricks for Tea Bags' examines the ways in which prostitution in institutions has gone largely unrecognised and unreported.

The third section highlights the links between the mental health system and the criminal justice system. There is an account by Julie McNamara of being forcibly detained and locked up by the police under Section 136 of the Mental Health Act, 1983. This section also includes the story of Josie O'Dwyer, a woman who did not survive the criminal justice system.

There are many issues that this chapter cannot cover in depth, including abuse by omission, for example the treatment of women with children in mental health services. It has been estimated that 40 per cent of women who use mental health services have or have had children. A study in West Lambeth found that 58 per cent of women using out-patient services were mothers, and many of those women have had their children forcibly removed. The study also found that there had been a lack of recognition about what this separation meant both for the women and their children (Iddamalgoda and Naish n.d.). The ways in which the experiences of lesbians, of Black women and older women have been pathologised or ignored also require close scrutiny if the services are to be seen as truly about care rather than containment and control.

We end the chapter by acknowledging the important gains that have been made in increasing choice for survivors but also by questioning if an individual 'consumer'-led response will really resolve the issue of abuse in the mental health system.

A culture of abuse?

Accounts of survivors suggest that we need to address the culture within which decisions are made in order to understand issues of abuse. Under the Mental Health Act, 1983, patients can be detained for up to six months on a Section 3 and forced to accept treatment whilst on section. British law allows for compulsory treatment, even when someone is not incapacitated, if they suffer from a mental disorder and it allows for six-month compulsory treatment sections, even though incapacity often only lasts hours or days. The legal framework surrounding treatment and detention without consent is an ever present part of the culture in mental health settings. In considering revisions to the Mental Health Act, 1983, discussions have been taking place on extending compulsory treatment orders to apply to people in the community (Bracken and Thomas 1998).

In 1997, three women spoke on television about their experiences in different psychiatric hospitals in the UK (*Over the Edge* 1997). Although each story was different, they had many similarities, and the following section draws from their stories amongst others.

Linda Ward entered the psychiatric system as a result of her relationship with her father:

> I first heard my father's voice when I was 9 years old. It said 'watch out. I'm watching you. I'm going to get you.' I didn't hear it again until years later. It became much more insistent and that led to me being taken into hospital, sectioned and drugged.
>
> (Linda, *Over the Edge* 1997)

Women enter the psychiatric system for a whole range of reasons, often involving abuse, neglect, loss and poverty (Brown and Harris 1978; Beck *et al.* 1987). For Terry Bailey, a series of losses precipitated her contact with the psychiatric system. She had lost a son and a daughter through cot deaths, and a cousin died (of cot death) while in her care:

> I couldn't shake the feeling I was to blame, even though the coroner explained that nothing could have been done. I went to my GP, frightened of what I would do. My feelings were so very intense. No one seemed to want to do anything. I knew I was

going to start a fire. I didn't know where I was going to do it or how. I bought some lighter fuel. I was walking; I came across a clothes shop for baby clothes, prams and cots. It seemed perfect.

(Terry, *Over the Edge* 1997)

Admission

Hospitalisation itself is a humiliating and dehumanising process. For patients taken in on a section, or through the criminal justice system, the process itself can be terrifying. On entering the hospital the patient is usually required to remove clothing and change into nightwear; personal effects are logged and taken away and she is allocated a bed or bedroom. This ritual alone is infantilising and de-personalising:

> When you go in on a section you are put in a nightdress with a great big flap that opens through the middle of the back: so you are not feeling well, not able to cope and you are going round the wards with your backside hanging out. Why in a mental hospital they have to have that type of gown (it's not a surgical ward) I really don't know.
>
> (Hall 1997)

Often women enter hospital experiencing disorientation and expecting some respite from emotional chaos but the environment itself is frightening and chaotic:

> After the fire, all of that chaos was gone; I was very calm. I had committed an offence; I wasn't going to be punished for it. I was sent to hospital. ... There was this guy muttering to himself, another guy with his arms outstretched telling me that he was going to take away my pain. ... I was badly burned at the time. I could feel the chaos starting again inside me.
>
> (Terry, *Over the Edge* 1997)

Those who hope for some kind of asylum and support, may find that the reality is very different and brings its own problems.

> At last here is a person I could talk to about my problems. ... I was crying when I went in, another misfit come home to the fold. Booked in – taken to have a bath – all my clothes and other possessions taken away – the nurses observing and writing what

my actions are; straight away I stopped crying and showed nothing.

(Hall 1986)

The ward environment

The woman is dependent upon the staff to meet her basic needs. Verbal exhortations and moral punishments are used to persuade patients to accept medication: 'Just take the drugs, just smile ... they used to say to me: smile and you'll get out, and I didn't bloody well feel like smiling. I felt in a lot of pain' (Veronica, *We're Not Mad We're Angry* 1985).

Whilst some survivors do find drugs helpful, the lack of control over the kind of medication, the amounts of medication and the combinations can be terrifying, as well as the side effects: 'I couldn't think, couldn't talk properly. I was dribbling and I had that mental patient shuffle' (Kari Haslam, *Over the Edge* 1997). The risks of tardive dyskinesia, a condition similar to Parkinson's Disease caused by the older neuroleptic drugs, are between 10–20 per cent for younger patients and 40 per cent for people over sixty (Breggin 1991). In some cases this is not reversible.

Women are subject to the culture of the particular hospital in which they are confined and often encouraged to conform to stereotypes of a 'good girl' and a compliant woman to be considered well:

I started off by trying to explain that I was upset about what was happening in the world that was making me depressed. Their answer was that I should be making more of an effort with my appearance and a lot of stuff about losing weight, wearing make up, doing something with my hair.

(Linda, *We're Not Mad We're Angry* 1985)

The ward environment allows the individual little control:

It was a feeling of punishment: you were locked in like a prisoner, when you wanted to go for a walk it was called going on parole; you were only allowed a drink every two hours, when you were taking medication that makes your mouth dry.

(Linda, *Over the Edge* 1997)

Contact between staff and patients in hospital is often limited and geared to drug taking and control: 'It was ward policy for staff not to talk to patients for more than ten minutes at a time and then not to talk about emotional matters' (Linda, *Over the Edge* 1997).

In many mental health settings, the open expression of strong emotions is actively discouraged:

> You were encouraged to sit in the day room and knit or sew. That was okay. You could get a colouring book and were encouraged to draw rivers that would show calm. One of the things you learnt quickly was not to show emotion ... in order to let the emotions out women took to hurting themselves or bingeing.
>
> (Terry, *Over the Edge* 1997)

Moira Potier, a psychologist who gave evidence to the Ashworth inquiry, analysed abuse in Ashworth Hospital in terms of power relationships and systems of control. These included 'techniques of oppression', such as seclusion, emotional abuse and use of sexist, racist and homophobic language. She also identified 'techniques of suppression' that included withdrawal of 'privileges' such as denying access to a patient's own clothes, visitors or books, as well as over-medication, double standards, divulging confidential information, intimidation and dirty tricks (Potier 1993). All these were common practices in an institution within which users had little power. An atmosphere of coercion and power imbalances, such as those experienced by users at Ashworth Hospital, makes real consent difficult. Obviously, mental health services differ in their location, their cultures and the degree of coercion they employ, but many of the practices she describes are used across the mental health system.

Consent to treatment

Even when people are admitted voluntarily many do not know that they have the right to refuse treatment, or can find that right difficult to exercise. Cobb's survey of older women who had received ECT found that most of the women aged over 50 in the study who had agreed to have ECT had done so under pressure. The following was typical of comments made by many older women patients who had had ECT, technically with their consent:

> I was, what I believe is termed an informal patient. The ward sister and the registrar kept coming to me with the form. I told them I

did not want ECT. In the hospital environment under drugs it is difficult to withstand staff pressure.

(Cobb 1996)

Treatment normally requires consent, but in an environment where people who use the mental health system are stigmatised, their words carry less weight. Sayce challenges us to examine consent closely:

It is tempting to think that when someone consents to sex or indeed to treatment then no violence takes place. But if we see violence not only as an individual attack but as something more patterned – a way of securing and entrenching power – then the context in which consent takes place can make consent suspect.

(1997: 5)

Women may consent to sex, in an atmosphere of intimidation where they have 'given up' resisting, or consent to treatment, with the belief that the threat of section lies behind it.

Sayce draws on accounts of activists and survivors to explore re-victimisation. She draws parallels between the forced treatment experienced by women and the sexual harassment and abuse that have often brought them to mental health services in the first place:

Punching, hitting, stabbing: we probably all think these are acts of violence and we would probably agree on groping (against a women's will), molesting, raping. If the key is that it is a physical and unwanted act committed on another person then forced injec-tions, forced ECT, forced feeding also seem to fit the bill: and it is noticeable that many women service users when asked about violence in mental health settings, speak as quickly of force in treatments, as they do of sexual or other physical assault.

If being in a mental institution can bring repeat experiences of sexual assault, being diagnosed mentally ill also adds a new layer of difficulty for women users: they have radically lost status and credibility and everything they say tends to be seen in terms of their illness. They become 'legitimate victims'. Whilst sexual assault might be dismissed, forced treatment is rarely seen by staff as assault at all.

Often this is because of a belief that treatment is beneficial: and if a woman becomes incapacitated, i.e. unable to understand what she might be consenting to and/or unable to weigh up the issue and make a choice, then someone needs to select the beneficial option on her behalf. Unfortunately this assessment of what is beneficial, whilst often positively motivated, rarely takes account of the fact that many women experience forced treatment as violence and betrayal.

(1997: 3–4)

The following is an extract from a letter received by the Women and Mental Health Network when readers were asked for contributions about violence in mental health services:

I was a user during the period June 1990 to October 1993 and experienced assaults both verbal and physical from both staff and patients in a Mental Health Unit. During my first admission I was frog marched back to my room, my arms twisted behind my back and I was held down in a horizontal position on the bed by two male staff nurses who trussed my legs up behind me like a chicken and I was given an injection in my buttocks. I was stark naked. Also my Consultant Psychiatrist threatened me with force if I refused to continue taking the drugs they had prescribed, on discharge.

(Anon. 1997)

For women who have experienced previous sexual abuse or rape, the experience of forced treatment and common institutional practices can be a further trauma. Jennings (1994) has drawn useful parallels between the events that led women into mental health services and the practices that re-victimise within the mental health system (see Table 7.1 on p. 163). Abuse is emotional as well as physical, and a number of survivors speak of the undermining of their confidence and individuality, of learning to be good and playing the game.

Sexual harassment and assault

Sexual harassment in mental health settings is an everyday occurrence. The number of women directly affected is not known, but MIND's Stress on Women campaign (Darton, Gorman and Sayce 1994) heard from women all over the country that they do not feel safe in mental health services.

Some talk of constant fear while, for example, being on a locked ward with men, others choose not to use services because of the

Table 7.1 Re-victimisation within psychiatric services

	Early childhood trauma	*Common institutional practice*
Trapped	Unable to escape perpetrators' abuse	Unable to escape institutional abuse. Locked up
Sexually violated	Stripped by abuser 'with nothing on below' Boundaries violated. Exposed, no privacy	To inject with medication, patient's pants pulled down, exposing buttocks and thighs, often by male attendants. No privacy from patients or staff. No boundaries
Isolated	Taken by abuser to places hidden from others	Forced, often by male attendants, into seclusion room
Unseen and unheard	Attempts to tell adults met with denial and silencing	Reports of past and present abuses interpreted as delusional
Blamed and shamed	'I had this feeling that I was bad ... a bad seed'	Patients stigmatised as deficient, mentally ill, worthless. Institutional practices convey low regard, tear down self worth
Threatened	As a child constant threat of being sexually violated	As a mental patient, constant threat of being stripped, thrown in seclusion, restrained, over medicated
Betrayal	Violated by trusted caretakers and relative	Retraumatised by helping professions

Source: Taken from Jennings (1994: 4).

abuse they or women they know, have experienced. Some women do not know they have a right not to be abused. Some keep quiet about abuse they have experienced because they are afraid they will not be believed or will be blamed.

(Wood and Copperman 1996)

The everyday ward experience can be intimidating for women:

The environment tends to be male dominated – the football is very loud on the TV, the radio is loud, the men are yelling to each other

– perhaps about a female body – and if you say something one of the excuses will be that the man is ill. You think to yourself what the hell am I in here for? … That is all they have to do, to stand there with a certain attitude, a certain look that is hard to explain even when you are well, but as a female you know that every portion of your body has been alerted by it.

(Hall 1997)

Problems do not only arise from the behaviour of other patients; some male staff specifically target women who are vulnerable and whose word would not easily be believed; for instance, Henry Bannerman was found guilty of two rapes in 1996, one against an older woman with drink problems and one against a woman with a diagnosis of schizophrenia whom he picked up in the corridors of Severalls Hospital in Essex (Sayce and Copperman 1997). A US study found that 38 per cent of residents in a psychiatric hospital had been sexually assaulted, and of these 27 per cent had suffered serious harassment or sexual assault by a staff member (Nibert *et al.* 1989). Below is a description of one woman's recent experience in a hospital in London:

When you are sectioned you can be put under very close one-to-one monitoring. That could be from a male nurse. I feel that this counts as sexual harassment – for instance, when my period started I had to go with this man into the toilet. They did not have sanitary towels, so in front of a male nurse who I didn't know, I had to change with toilet paper.

(Hall 1997)

There is little control over this sexually threatening environment:

I was locked up for a year in hospital with a man who constantly harassed me. This man still harasses me on the streets. I am frightened of him knowing my address. I have fought him off. I was also sexually harassed by a male nurse. This male nurse used to come into my room and say to me, 'Come on then, come and get me and I will have you on the bed.' Then when I did eventually go for him, he would put me on the bed, he would ring up the team and hurt me.

(Hall 1997)

Redress

Complaints often go unheard or become lost in bureaucracy. In one study of users of mental health services (Lewisham Black Mental Health Association 1991), a 16-year-old woman reported having been raped by one of the night staff in hospital. Her experience of reporting abuse is not uncommon. When, next morning, she told her mother what had happened, it was reported to the day nurse. The doctor came and told her mother that it was part of her daughter's illness: she was fantasising. The incident was not formally recorded, no investigation took place and the woman ended up creating a disturbance, so she was placed on a locked ward out of the man's reach. In response to her report of the assault, she was given higher doses of medication and locked up.

Even when policies and procedures are in place, there can be a reluctance to publicise and implement them. One patients' council reported that it took over a year to get a notice on the door of the relevant manager and to get the policy disseminated to the wards (Communicate 1998). There is within the context of mental health services a frequent disbelief of survivors' voices and a routine denial that abuse took place – 'it's all part of her illness' – together with claims that the woman consented. Blame is also used to deny the reality of abuse: 'when she is ill she gets very manipulative'. This complaint was finally upheld but not without a struggle:

> It took me nine months to find out there was a procedure I could go through; and it was not until I came out that I felt brave enough to act … it takes a lot of courage to complain, because when you complain they still have control over you. If you talk to a nurse you are talking about their colleague. They can forcibly inject you, you have the label as mad, you are frightened, everything is working against you. He had started doing the same things to somebody else. The complaints procedure was meant to take twenty days; it took three months.
>
> (Hall 1997)

Although an assurance was finally given by the hospital that this nurse in question would not be left alone with women in the future this advice was ignored and further complaints ensued.

Prostitution

Prostitution in residential-care settings has been an unexplored area of emotional abuse in institutional settings. One study found that, out of fifty-three women in-patients, 56 per cent had been pestered, including being touched on the legs, breasts and bottom, and being constantly asked to have sex, while 12 per cent of the women had been asked to have sex for favours, including cigarettes, money or alcohol (unpublished study cited in London Borough of Southwark 1996).

> Prostitution is rife amongst women within residential care settings and particularly amongst women who are emotionally vulnerable. ... Women who behave like 'good girls' and comply with their treatment will be allowed access to their money. Women who do not comply are denied their money and then have no access to the comforts that make life in hospital a little more bearable.
>
> To earn comforts such as extra tea, sweets and cigarettes they may be subjected to pressure from male patients, visitors and staff to provide sexual favours. It is men within hospital settings who have the strangle hold on this subculture of prostitution for peanuts.
>
> In 'secure' settings women may be left at the mercy of organised prostitution syndicates. Or women become prey to the lone males hovering around residential care settings ready to 'court' vulnerable women and offer them ciggies for sex.
>
> (McNamara and Radclyffe 1997: 8)

It is tempting to think that with the shift towards smaller institutions that these problems will dissipate but anecdotal evidence suggests that women remain vulnerable to these pressures.

The mental health system, criminal justice and abuse

The use of the criminal justice system to deal with mental distress has been the focus of considerable concern by survivors. Section 136 of the Mental Health Act, 1983 gives the police powers to detain someone they consider a danger to themselves or a danger to the public. This power is often used loosely and applied unequally. The preponderance of Black people picked up in this area on Section 136 has been highlighted, and the lack of clear procedures or training for police officers has been identified. The following account highlights the violent treatment received by Julie McNamara, one of the authors of this chapter, after an incident in a therapeutic environment.

> I had had a period of six months away from my post, trying to deal with the shock of six bereavements in quick succession. After counselling I had decided to go into a crisis centre.
>
> (McNamara 1997: 13)

The contrasts between the emotional support she was hoping for on entering a therapeutic setting and the reality that ensued are stark:

> On 5 March 1994 one of the residents at the clinic slashed his wrist in the art therapy session. The events of the day spiralled out of control after the art therapist went home.
>
> Junior members of staff were left in charge, horror videos and alcohol were brought into the centre, finally events got out of hand.
>
> I flipped and put my head through some of the windows. I am told that I hit a therapist during a struggle. I hid in a bush in the garden, he panicked and rang for the police. I was taken in handcuffs and ankle restraints on my belly in the back of the police van. I was seized by six police officers from the grounds of the crisis centre on Section 136, roughed up in the van, imprisoned for four hours and then taken off to St. Ann's lock-in facility. My body was covered in bruises and I bore the mark of a jack boot on my back for weeks following. The violence with which I was treated shocked me to the core.
>
> None of the officers in attendance had any experience in mental health. I was not accompanied by anybody trained in mental health from the clinic. My rights were not read, I was refused access to a telephone and most of my clothes were removed.
>
> (McNamara 1997: 13)

These procedures as well as being terrifying also leave the recipient with a police record.

Many of the most vulnerable women end up in the criminal justice system in medium secure units or in special hospitals. Women in Prison estimate that two-thirds of the women in prison have been sexually abused in childhood (WISH 1997) and that over 70 per cent of the women in Special Hospitals have been sexually abused in childhood (WISH 1997). The criminal justice system overall has shown little understanding of mental distress. In 1998, the prison inspectorate walked out of the women's psychiatric unit in Holloway prison in protest at the appalling conditions that it found there.

Continuing abuse can have devastating consequences, as in the case of Josie O'Dwyer. Like many women in prison, she was abused in childhood and grew up in care. She was convicted in 1995 of murdering a man who was trying to rape her. Against the advice of her lawyers she pleaded guilty to a charge of murder, which carries a life sentence, after having heard in open court that she herself had been abused as a child by her father, a memory she had disassociated from and that caused her to have an epileptic seizure. The judge refused to adjourn the session to allow her time to absorb and deal with this information. Terrified of being 'nutted off' – i.e. sent to one of the Special Hospitals – she chose instead to plead guilty to murder. Over-medication and a prescribed cocktail of drugs are common in prison environments; in Josie O'Dwyer's case she committed suicide in prison after two years. Eleven different drugs that were being taken simultaneously appeared on her drug sheet when she died. It took three hours for help to arrive after her suicide attempt was discovered (*Channel 4 News* 1998). This might be an extreme case but it illustrates some of the consequences of a lifetime of unchecked institutional abuse.

Conclusion

In drawing together the accounts of women survivors it has been difficult to believe that society has been guilty of such unimaginative responses to women in distress. Far worse is the realisation that these voices of unrest have often gone unheard and the testimonies of women complainants discounted.

There have been positive changes: survivor voices are becoming stronger, either through the establishment of user-run services such as the Sanctuary in Brixton, or through inclusion in the planning of services, for example, user representation on the Government's national mental health task force. Too often, however, the underlying patterns of power and powerlessness remain untouched and users wield little real power in these forums.

The closure of large hospitals has also opened up the possibility of establishing pioneering services like the women's crisis house in Camden and Islington, which makes provision for women and their children and the 24-hour crisis service for women with mental health problems and a history of abuse in Birmingham. But these are isolated examples of good practice, and the smaller residential settings in which many users find themselves within do not necessarily represent a change in culture from the large hospitals they replace. Women in institutional care need access to a safe environment, supportive care and the redress that comes from independent scrutiny.

The culture of discrediting the testimonies of women who have been diagnosed as 'mentally ill' is gradually being challenged and the reality of abuse recognised. Some trusts have revised their complaints procedures to take account of sexual and other forms of abuse, and have developed specific policies and procedures to deal with them. For example, the Maudsley Hospital, Pathfinder Trust and Southampton City Council have drawn up policies and procedures on reporting and dealing with abuse that ensure that it is taken more seriously, but it has often been difficult to back policies up with resources and training. How can it be ensured that, within the existing culture, where 'rivers of abuse' exist these policies do not remain paper policies and are implemented and backed up with training and support for users who do complain? Will the Crown Prosecution Service change its reluctance to prosecute in cases of alleged rape because a woman has a diagnosis of mental illness?

Campaigns on certain issues of individual choice have met with some success: for example, in 1995, the Patient's Charter stated that women should expect single-sex washing and toilet facilities, and should be informed if they were being admitted to mixed or single-sex facilities. In 1998, directives have been issued to health authorities to reinforce this but many women, like those in Special Hospitals and medium secure units, still do not have access to a safe environment.

Many questions remain to be answered. Will the same patterns of oppression be carried over into many of the smaller institutions that survivors find themselves within? What of the disbelief that is still accorded to survivors when they do experience abuse? Continued hostility to users of mental health services is evident in many quarters in the debates about community care.

It remains the case that public funding has been supporting a system of mental health care that has behaved more like the strong arm of social control, containing and controlling rather than supporting the most vulnerable members of society. At a policy and planning level, the unequal structures of power that leave women in distress with so few civil rights or little dignity have to be challenged. Strategies of intervention need to be redesigned in response to the evidence of those survivors' voices. Care packages that take account of women's social and economic position in their own communities have more relevance than the chemical coshes offered within many mental health services. The aftermath of sexual abuse and rape, of poverty and deprivation cannot be cured by chemical strait jackets, seclusion or detention without trial, which is what many mental health systems offer.

Vulnerable women need respite in their own communities, with access to good-quality childcare, support networks, choices of treatment, access to talking treatments, full information about available medication and alternative treatments. Finally, women need the support to be able to regain control of their own lives. If we are to advance from a system that is ultimately failing its users, women's voices must be heard.

References

Anon. (1997) Letter, *Women and Mental Health Forum Newsletter* 3, September: 17.

Bean, P., Bingley, W., Bynoe, I., Faulkner, A., Rassaby, E. and Rogers, A. (1991) *Out of Harm's Way*, London: MIND.

Beck, J.C. and Van, D.K.B. (1987) 'Reports of childhood incest and current behaviour of chronically hospitalized psychotic women', *American Journal of Psychiatry* 144(11): 1474–6.

Blom-Cooper, L. (1992) *Report of the Committee of Inquiry into Complaints about Ashworth Hospital*, vols 1 and 2, Cmd 2028-1, London: HMSO.

Bouhoustos, J., Holroyd, J., Lerman, H., Forer, B. and Greenberg, M. (1983) 'Sexual intimacies between psychotherapists and patients', *Professional Psychology: Research and Practice* 14: 185–96.

Bracken, P. and Thomas, P. (1998) 'Mental health legislation: Time for a real change', *OpenMind* 98, March/April: 17.

Breggin, P. (1991) *Toxic Psychiatry*, London: St Martin's Press.

Brown, G.W. and Harris, T. (1978) *Social Origins of Depression*, London: Tavistock Publications.

Channel 4 News (1998) 'Item on drugs and women in hospital', 28 October.

Cobb, A. (1996) *Older Women and ECT*, London: MIND.

Communicate (1998) Personal communication, London: Patients' Group, Maudsley Hospital.

Cutting Edge (1991) 'A special hospital', 4 March (Channel 4).

Darton, K., Gorman, J. and Sayce, L. (1994) *Eve Fights Back: Successes of MIND's Stress on Women Campaign*, London: MIND.

Dundas, D.W. (1995) 'The shocking truth', in J. Grobe (ed.) (1995) *Beyond Bedlam*, Chicago: Third Side Press.

Eastman, N. (1995) 'Anti-therapeutic community mental health law', *British Medical Journal* 310: 10,811–12.

Edwardes, M. and Fasal, J. (1992) 'Keeping an intimate relationship professional', *OpenMind* 57: 10–11.

Faulkner, A. (1996) *Knowing Our Own Minds*, London: Mental Health Foundation.

Garrett, T. (1992) *Summary of Findings of a National Survey of Clinical Psychologists with Reference to Sexual Contact with Patients*, report available from POPAN, London.

Hall, M. (1997) 'Interview with Jeanette Copperman', *Women and Mental Health Forum Newsletter* 3, September: 11–12.

Hall, S. (1986) 'I've seen pink and white fairies dancing on bushes', in P. McNeill, M. McShea and P. Parmar (eds) *Through The Break*, London: Sheba Press.

Iddamalgoda, K. and Naish, J. (n.d.) *Nobody Cared about Me*, London: West Lambeth Community Health Trust.

Ingram, R. (1993) *Violence from Known Men: Women and Mental Health*, unpublished paper, Leeds Interagency Project.

Jennings, A. (1994) 'On being invisible in the mental health system', *Journal of Mental Health Administration* 21: 4.

Lewisham Black Mental Health Association (1991), interview with researcher.

Liverpool Daily Post (1997), 8 November.

London Borough of Southwark (1996) *Draft Strategy for Women's Mental Health*, unpublished.

McNamara, J. (1996) 'Out of order: Madness is a feminist and a disability issue', in J. Morris (ed.) *Encounters With Strangers*, London: Women's Press.

—— (1997) 'Shock tactics', *Women and Mental Health Forum Newsletter* 3, September: 13–15.

McNamara, J. and Radclyffe, K. (1998) 'Turning tricks for tea bags', *Women and Mental Health Forum Newsletter* 4, May: 8–9.

MIND (1992) *The Hidden Majority*, London: MIND Publications.

Multiple Image (1985) *We're Not Mad We're Angry*, video, London: Mental Health Media.

Nibert, C., Cooper, S. and Crossmaker, M. (1989) 'Assaults against residents of a psychiatric institution', *Journal of Interpersonal Violence* 4: 342–9.

Over The Edge (1997) 'Sectioned', 17 September (BBC2).

Potier, M. (1993) 'Giving evidence: Women's lives in Ashworth Maximum Security Psychiatric Hospital', *Feminism and Psychology* 3(3): 335–47.

Rogers, A., Pilgrim, D. and Lacey, R. (1993) *Experiencing Psychiatry*, London: MIND.

Sainsbury Centre (1997) *The National Visit: A One Day Visit to 309 Acute Psychiatric Wards*, London: Sainsbury Centre for Mental Health.

Sayce, L. (1997) 'Voices not just choices: Extending our challenges to violence in mental health settings', *Women and Mental Health Forum Newsletter* 3, September: 3–8.

Sayce, L. and Copperman, J. (1997) 'Violence against women in mental health settings', *Women and Mental Health Forum Newsletter* 3, September: 1–3.

Wallcraft, J. and Read, J. (1994) *Guidelines on Advocacy for Mental Health Workers*, London: Unison Health Care/MIND.

Williams, J. and Watson, G. (1994) 'Mental health services that empower women: The challenge to clinical psychology', *Clinical Psychology Forum* 64: 6–12.

Williams, J., Watson, G., Smith, H., Copperman, J. and Wood, D. (1993) *Purchasing Effective Mental Health Services for Women: A Framework for Action*, Canterbury: University of Kent.

WISH (Women in Special Hospitals) (1997) *Annual Report: Listening to Women, a Force for Change*, London: WISH (Women in Special Hospitals).

Wood, D. and Copperman, J. (1996) *Sexual Harassment and Assault in Psychiatric Services*, London: Good Practices in Mental Health.

8 The abuse of older people in institutional settings

An overview

Frank Glendenning

In the 1970s and 1980s investigators in the US sought to establish and clarify our understanding of elder abuse and neglect. The case material that they used was recognisable elsewhere as well. But because it was largely concerned with domestic settings, we became dependent in our description of elder abuse and neglect on the family violence model. Surprisingly, little work was done in the US during that period on the abuse and neglect of older people in institutional settings. Not until Pillemer's work in the US, and Clough's work in Britain in the 1980s, did findings of major significance for our understanding of abuse and neglect in institutions begin to emerge. Now, additionally in the last few years, it has become apparent that we are confronted with an international problem in both domestic and institutional settings (Kosberg and Garcia 1995; Glendenning and Kingston 1999). But overall, there is an absence of reliable prevalence studies.

Whilst the extent of abuse in informal or family settings is very unclear, its existence within institutions in Britain has been widely documented (Phillipson and Biggs 1995: 189). Townsend published *The Last Refuge* in 1962, Robb reported on hospitals (*Sans Everything: A Case to Answer*) in 1967 as did Martin in *Hospitals in Trouble* in 1984. Willcocks *et al.* reported on residential homes in the public sector in 1986 (see also Peace *et al.* 1997). In 1988, at the invitation of the Wagner Committee on Residential Care, Clough presented a report on *Scandals in Residential Homes*. This was never published. Holmes and Johnson wrote about private homes in 1988. In 1989, Horrocks analysed Health Advisory Service reports on long-stay wards in hospitals (cited in Tomlin 1989: 11) and the Harman sisters reported on the first ninety-six cases considered under the 1984 Registered Homes Act. Counsel and Care reported on privacy and restraint in 1991 and 1992, and on abuse in care homes in 1995.

When discussing this subject, it has been customary to draw a distinction between individual acts of abuse in institutions and actual institutional or institutionalised abuse (Glendenning 1997: 151). As Decalmer (1993: 59) has suggested, abuse of the person is common, but the commonest abuse of all is institutional abuse, where the environment, practices and rules of the institution become abusive in themselves, a view underscored by Peace *et al.* (1997: 67). This being so, how with our existing knowledge about elder abuse should we proceed in relation to our search for strategies to prevent it?

The changing picture

A number of investigators have attempted to quantify the changes that have taken place in residential care during the last twenty-five years. Higgs and Victor have shown that between 1970 and 1990, the number of residential places in British institutions nearly doubled, reaching nearly half a million places, with over 200,000 being in the independent sector. More recently, Peace *et al.* have set out the figures up to 1994 (1997: 21). They indicate that the total number of places in 1970 was 247,300 of which 83,000 were in the independent sector.

Then, from 1980, Supplementary Benefit offices were given discretion under the Supplementary Regulations (Regulation 9) to use their discretion to pay board and lodging allowances to older people in private-care homes that were 'reasonable'. This doubled the number of claimants between 1980 and 1983. The annual cost rose from £18 million in 1980 to £5.5 billion in 1990 (Higgs and Victor 1993: 190).

Peace *et al.* demonstrate that the numbers of residential places rose to 536,000 in 1994, 413,000 of which were in the independent sector. They further suggest that the cost of residential care in 1995 stood at £8 billion per annum, of which the private sector share was £4.6 billion (Peace *et al.* 1997: 21–5). Regarding this as evidence of a new cottage industry, Peace *et al.* remark that, between 1981 and 1991, the residential population grew at a much faster rate than the older population itself and 'this suggests that an explanation for the increase in numbers of homes is likely to lie somewhere between political ideology and demographics' (1997: 15).

Studies and findings in the United States

It may be helpful to set out here some of the principal work that has been reported during the last few years. As long ago as 1973 in the United States, Stannard published a paper in *Social Problems* entitled 'Old folks and dirty work'. In his observation study of a nursing home, he identified slapping, hitting, shaking a patient, pulling hair, tightening restraining belts and terrorising by gesture and word (Stannard 1973).

In the 1980s and 1990s, a number of studies focused on the quality of life in residential homes. Kimsey *et al.*, for example, examined 1,000 nursing homes in Texas in 1981 and found that, while physical abuse was less common, physical neglect was far more apparent and psychological abuse was frequent wherever there was passive neglect (1981: 465). Tarbox published a paper in 1983 on the psychological aspects of neglect in nursing homes. He emphasised the lack of cleanliness and attractiveness in the physical environment, inadequate diet, infantilisation and passive neglect (Tarbox 1983: 42–6).

In 1983, Doty and Sullivan studied the statistics of the Federal Certification Agency and concluded that a significant proportion of institutions were assessed as being 'deficient on the requirement that each patient is treated with consideration, respect and full dignity'. When in the same year, they studied nursing homes in New York, they found evidence of over-medication and insanitary conditions, and that patients who could not feed themselves were not being fed (1983: 223–4).

There had been a scandal in 1980 over Medicaid fraud in the United States and in 1983, Halamandaris, a senior lawyer, published his findings and listed a cavalcade of abuse in American nursing homes: theft from patients' funds, false claims by carers to both Medicare and Medicaid, trading in real estate, fraudulent therapy and pharmaceutical charges, even involvement in organised crime (1983: 104–14).

Again, in 1983, Stathopoulos reported on an advocacy service in North Central Massachusetts that was compelled to develop strategies in order to deal with financial abuse, denial of civil rights and various kinds of maltreatment in nursing homes. The principal goal was to improve the quality of care in homes and to alter the power equilibrium in favour of residents or consumers. The training of volunteer advocates and the importance of networking were among its priorities (1983: 336–54).

Similarly, Solomon, who investigated the pharmacological and non-pharmacological abuse of elderly patients, concluded that care staff were poorly trained and had an extremely high turnover. In his view the frustrations of the job could lead to the infantilisation, derogation and actual physical abuse of patients (1983: 159).

In 1990, Fader *et al.* published their study of health care workers in long-term settings in New York and the way in which the workers perceived elder abuse in relation to active and passive neglect. Their testing demonstrated that nurse aides had significantly lower scores than licensed practical nurses. They concluded that 'there must be ongoing education and training about abuse and neglect' (1990: 89; see also Foner 1994).

In 1990, also, Wiener and Kayser-Jones published a paper about the interaction of nursing-home staff with patients and relatives. They showed that both staff and patients/relatives had complaints concerning each other: the staff complained about being short-staffed and the sense that they were not working as a team, with a lack of resources such as sheets, towels and simple ointments (1990: 95).

Maltreatment in nursing homes

While therefore there was no lack of awareness about the general problem of mistreatment in residential settings, apart from the Texas study we did not have a thorough review of maltreatment in nursing homes until Pillemer (1988) and Pillemer and Moore (1989, 1990). Pillemer revisited his study with Bachman-Prehn (1991) and with Lachs (1995). Although mentioned briefly by McCreadie (1991) in her study of abuse in domestic settings, Pillemer's findings were not widely accessible in Britain until Bennett and Kingston obtained permission to publish some of them in 1993. Their conclusion was that when Pillemer and Moore's evidence was set alongside the evidence of the British official inquiry reports, it may be that, as Pillemer has indicated, abuse in institutions is relatively widespread (Bennett and Kingston 1993: 125–6). Further references to Pillemer's study may be found in other British texts: Phillipson and Biggs (1992: 173; 1995: 191–2); Glendenning (1993: 13–14; 1996: 41–3; 1997: 155–60) [In the latter, Pillemer's theoretical model of patient maltreatment is visually presented and discussed (p.160)]; McCreadie (1996: 58–62).

Pillemer and Moore, in undertaking their study in 1987, were conscious that it was problematic to establish prevalence figures for abuse and neglect in nursing homes. Monk *et al.* had already reported in 1984 that over half the nursing-home residents who were interviewed in their sample said they had refrained from making a complaint for fear of reprisals. This led Pillemer and Moore to decide to conduct a random survey of nursing-home staff in one state, and to publish their findings fully (Pillemer 1988; Pillemer and Moore 1989, 1990). We have noted already that several investigators in Britain have described their findings and there is little to be gained by repeating these descriptions at length here. In summary, Pillemer and Moore worked with a sample of 577 nurses and nursing aides drawn from thirty-two homes, which ranged in size from 19 to 300 beds. Telephone interviews were conducted in Spring 1987. They examined the issue of the extent of abuse and the causes of maltreatment within the general context of nursing-home care by building up a profile of staff and confining their investigation to skilled nursing facilities (which provided 24-hour care) and to intermediate-care nursing homes (where intensive care was not required but where patients had functional impairments). 'Staff' were defined as registered nurses, licensed practical nurses and nursing aides.

They found that:

- the average length of employment in the home was less than five years;
- the average length of total employment was seven-and-a-half years;
- the average age (ranging from 16 to 64) was 40;
- there were high levels of job stress (lack of time being given as one reason);
- nearly half reported that fewer staff turned up than were scheduled on three or more days a week;
- based on responses to Maslach's burn-out inventory (1982), they found high levels of burn-out that was strongly related to stress;
- 36 per cent of the sample had seen at least one incident of physical abuse during the preceding year;
- 70 per cent had seen staff yelling at patients;
- 10 per cent admitted that they themselves had committed such actions;
- 6 per cent had used excessive restraint;
- 40 per cent had committed at least one act of psychological abuse during the preceding year;
- 13 per cent reported denying food or privileges.

This catalogue of self-reported abuse is alarming by any standard, but Pillemer and Moore suggested that some under-reporting of negative actions had probably occurred and although these estimates could not be compared with others that were compatible, they believed that there was sufficiently extensive evidence of abuse to merit concern (Pillemer and Moore 1989: 314–20). Separate statistical analyses were made to identify predictors of negative actions, paying attention to staff–patient conflict and level of burn-out (see also Pillemer and Bachman-Prehn 1991).

This extremely important study concluded that well-qualified staff did not choose to work in nursing homes, where work is physically taxing, wages are poor and job prestige low. Ways of reducing stress were seen to be a major priority for administrators and training needs were also seen to be critical for the management of patients' behaviour and aggression. Working in situations of very high conflict, staff themselves run serious risk of verbal and physical assault by patients, a point reiterated in the findings of a study in Bristol (Eastley *et al.* 1993) and also in a recent Canadian study (Goodridge *et al.* 1996).

Pillemer and Moore found that 27 per cent of staff had conflicts every day over patients' unwillingness to eat, and 26 per cent said that they had this kind of conflict a few times a week. Similar high rates were found to occur over patients' personal hygiene, dressing and toileting. Ninety per cent of staff had been subject to insults or swearing during the previous year; 50 per cent more than ten times. Forty-seven per cent had been kicked or bitten by patients during the previous year, and in 11 per cent of cases this had happened ten or more times. Pillemer and Moore remarked that verbal aggression and even physical violence appears to be one of the basic features of nursing-home life. As a result of this data we can build a picture of high staff stress in comparison with the experience of almost any other profession.

The quality of care in nursing homes was shown to have been better in homes that could afford to hire staff with better training and where staff–patient ratios were relatively high. High staff turnover rates could be correlated with poor quality care. Nurses and nursing aides with lower levels of education were likely to have more negative attitudes towards older people.

Improving staff training

The major outcome of this study was an endeavour to improve staff training. Together with Hudson and others, Pillemer developed a model abuse prevention programme for nursing assistants called *Ensuring an Abuse-Free Environment* (CARIE (Coalition of Advocates for the Rights of Infirm Elders) 1991; see Pillemer and Hudson 1993 and Keller 1996). In this way, they underscored the necessity of upgrading the quality of long-term nursing-home care. This model programme is made up of eight modules written in non-technical language, including reflection on being a professional caregiver, definitions and indicators of abuse, strategies for defusing potentially abusive situations, conflict management skills and techniques. It includes a technique called RETHINK that provides a step-by-step approach to dealing with conflict (Keller 1996: 236; see also Decalmer 1997: 53). Pillemer and Moore's conviction that it is essential to improve staff training has since been confirmed by British research (Baillon *et al.* 1996: 225). Pillemer and Moore emphasise that inappropriate management practice and staff–patient interaction require further study. Certainly, staff screening and development are required to protect patients and ways must be found of reducing the stress experienced by staff. Keller has described how the implementation of the CARIE abuse prevention programme resulted in a decline of self-reported abusive incidents (Keller 1996: 238).

In the late 1950s, Erving Goffman, when he was at the US National Institute of Mental Health, conducted a year's participant study at St Elizabeth's Hospital, Washington, DC and as a result wrote his famous text, *Asylums*, which was first published in 1961. In his essay, 'On the Characteristics of Total Institutions', he wrote:

> Many total institutions, most of the time, seem to function merely as storage dumps for inmates ... but they usually present themselves to the public as rational organizations designed consciously, through and through, as effective machines for producing a few officially avowed and officially approved ends.
>
> (Goffman 1968: 73)

We need to bear this thought in mind when we come to discuss later the attitude of the establishment towards scandals and abuse in particular institutions.

Residential care in the UK

While these studies in the United States had been going on, laying out some of the principal reasons why maltreatment occurs in residential situations, and making recommendations for improved management and staff training, Roger Clough in Britain had from the 1970s made a major contribution to our understanding of residential care. His book, *Old Age Homes*, was published in 1981. In it, he emphasised the rights and choices to which residents were entitled. As a social work teacher and later as a Chief Inspector of Social Services in the North West, he has always brought a unique clarity to his declared concern for the quality of care in residential homes. For example, quite recently, he wrote:

The cruelty that thrives on secrecy is how the *Independent* (1994) in a leading article described abuse in residential homes. How does it happen that in the very places where people have gone for care, they find themselves abused by others? At the centre of the concern about the abuse of people in residential homes and nursing homes lies a terrifying reality: in such homes, it is not possible to guarantee even the minimum that people will not be abused. It is tempting to use increasingly powerful words to describe the awfulness of such events. ... Yet constant repetition of the horrors may contribute little to the understanding either of the reasons how and why abuse occurs, or why abuse is not stopped.

(Clough 1996: 3; see also the chapter by Clough in this volume)

British boards of inquiry

In Britain, as a result of official boards of inquiry, episodes involving the ill-treatment of patients and poor standards of care in hospitals and residential homes are well documented, as Phillipson and Biggs (1995) have reminded us. In 1988, Clough was invited to submit evidence to the Wagner Committee on Residential Care. His report, *Scandals in Residential Centres*, was an analysis of some twenty of these public inquiry reports about abuse and neglect in care homes. It raised fundamental questions about the nature of residential institutions. For over a decade, these were frequently referred to by investigators through judicious leaks from the report, but the report itself remained unpublished. Extracts, however, were eventually published with the author's permission (Glendenning 1996: 44–6; 1997: 157–9).

At the beginning of his report, Clough reflected on what we had *not* learnt from the past and noted the public statement of David Ennals, a former Secretary for Social Services, who declared in 1979:

We have had a succession of public enquiries pointing up the grave inadequacies in public hospitals ... [but] little has changed for the better in some of them. ... I am determined that this gap between the good and the bad shall not remain as wide as it is today.

(cited in Clough 1988a)

But within eight years, there were two more reports. One illustrated the poor management of care homes for older people in Camden. The report, cited by Clough in 1988, concluded that 'effective management of residential care in Camden has broken down'. And the appalling report about pervasive abuse at Nye Bevan Lodge, Southwark, stated that there was:

> an atmosphere of deep mistrust and suspicion which [had] perme-
> ated every aspect of life in the home for many years resulting in a
> serious deterioration in the level of care provided [and] as such
> that a proper level of caring could never be restored given the
> same staff and officers.
>
> (cited in Clough 1988a)

Clough recorded that the actions of staff included neglecting to wash or bath residents and charging them for bathing, probably as a means of reducing the number of people to be bathed; punishing those who complained by leaving one resident's feet in excessively hot water for a long time; opening windows and removing blankets at night so that in consequence some caught pneumonia and died. Some residents were involved in falls following altercations with staff; the bar in the home was used by a few staff and outsiders who were noisy and sometimes molested staff or residents.

The Nye Bevan Lodge scandal aroused much public concern and one commentator wrote in *Nursing Times*:

> It is self-evident that when elderly, often confused residents are
> made to eat their own faeces, are left unattended, are physically
> man-handled or are forced to pay money to care staff and even
> helped to die, there is something seriously wrong.
>
> (Vousden 1987: 19)

It is therefore instructive to recognise that Wagner studiously avoided raising the implications of these notorious reports together with others of the 1970s and 1980s, together with Clough's reflections on them. The literature surveys that were attached as volume 2 of the Wagner report (Sinclair 1988) contain no reference to them either and we are left with the distinct impression that they were deliberately suppressed (Glendenning 1996: 27).

Nearly twenty years earlier, when R.H.S. Crossman became Secretary of State for Health and Social Services, he found that he had inherited an 83,000-word report, commissioned by the previous Minister of Health, into the criminal malpractices at the Ely Mental Hospital in Cardiff. Unknown to Crossman, according to his biogra-pher, Anthony Howard, officials in the Department had been conducting a six-month wrangle with the author of the report, the then young Tory barrister, Geoffrey Howe, over how little of his indictment they could get away with publishing. Although it meant overruling nearly all his civil servants, Crossman insisted on publishing the report in full, combined with the simultaneous announcement of a new system of inspectors, reporting direct to the Secretary of State for all learning disability, geriatric or psychiatric hospitals (Howard 1990: 295).

These are merely two examples of attempted misinformation over a period of twenty years. Wardhaugh and Wilding in reviewing a particular public inquiry report concerning the treatment of young people during the 1980s and writing about the corruption of care, commented:

> What is remarkable is that every level of management appears to have been guilty. Middle and senior management were equally contemptuous of complaints and dilatory in pursuing them. So were Hospital Management Committees, Regional Hospital Boards and the Department of Health and Social Security. As Dick Crossman's memoirs reveal (*Political Diaries*, vol. 3. 411), the Department knew about the unsatisfactory conditions at Ely Hospital [Cardiff] long before the Howe Report.
>
> (1993: 18–19)

Recalling the words of Goffman cited earlier, it is tempting to be cynical and say 'There is no new thing under the sun'! (Ecclesiastes 1: 9).

Lessons to be learnt

Clough put forward a number of explanations concerning what was to be learnt from the scandals in his report to the Wagner Committee:

- There was a failure within the managing agency to agree about purposes and tasks.
- There was a failure to manage life in the institutions in an appropriate way.
- There was a shortage of resources and staff.
- There was confusion and lack of knowledge and frequent absence of guidelines.
- There was the attitude and behaviour of staff, inadequate staffing levels and training and low staff morale.
- Low status was ascribed to the work.

- There was a failure to perceive a pattern in events, individual events being treated in isolation.

(1988a)

Clough also wrote more generally in one of the journals, that abuse of residents is more likely when:

> There have been a series of complaints over a long period, relating to more than one member of staff; the establishment is run down and basic arrangements for laundry and hygiene are poor, for example a pervasive smell of urine; there are staff shortages and staff sickness; senior staff are on holiday; there is little supervision of staff and they are able to develop their own patterns of work (we know little of what happens at night time); staff have been in charge of the unit for a considerable time; there is a high turnover of staff; staff drink alcohol regularly during breaks or when on duty; there is uncertainty about the future of the establishment; there are few visitors; residents are highly dependent on staff for personal care; residents go out little or have few contacts; a partic- ular resident has no-one taking an active interest in him or her; there is discord among the staff team or between staff and managers; the residents are troublesome, when their care makes heavy demands or when the task to be carried out is unpleasant.
> (Clough 1988b: 7; see also Clough, 1999, where he breaks the 1988 imposed silence for the first time)

Models of resident/patient maltreatment

Commenting on Clough's findings, Phillipson and Biggs (1995: 191) have suggested that they imply a model in which resident maltreatment is related to three key factors: (i) the home environment; (ii) staff char- acteristics; and (iii) patient/resident characteristics. In this they follow Pillemer (1988: 230), who first broached this as a provisional theoret- ical model of patient maltreatment and found it validated by his subsequent research (Glendenning 1997: 159–60). Pillemer also suggested in his model that there may be exogenous factors as well; for example, the supply and demand of hospital beds and the unemploy- ment rate, which may need to be taken into account. (This is discussed in more detail in Bennett and Kingston 1993: 118; Phillipson and Biggs 1992: 115–16; 1995: 192; Glendenning, 1997: 160.) Working independently on either side of the Atlantic Ocean, both Clough and Pillemer came to remarkably similar conclusions in the same year.

The Wagner Report on Residential Care in 1988, while omitting any reference to known abuse and neglect, nevertheless said that living in a residential establishment should be a positive experience ensuring a better quality of life than the resident could enjoy in any other setting, and that the contribution of staff should be recognised and enhanced.

Alternatively, in the last decade according to its annual reports, the UK Central Council for Nursing, Midwifery and Health Visiting (UKCC) has seen an increase in the number of reported cases of misconduct in the nursing-home sector, involving physical and psychological abuse, inadequate systems of drug administration and ineffective management systems. In 1994, it reported that nursing-home cases were nearly 100 per cent greater than any other area of practice (UKCC 1994: 1; see also Clough 1988b; 1996: 10–26; Ferguson 1996: 158–65). Hughes has suggested that 'institutions, because of their semi-closed environment and the intimate nature of care required, appear to be environments in which abuse can occur unreported and undetected for significant periods of time' (Hughes 1995: 136).

Abuse and neglect in hospitals

During the course of this chapter, we have discussed almost exclusively the situation in residential and nursing homes. But we should not ignore the fact that abuse and neglect of elderly people can take place in hospitals as well. The issue of elder abuse and neglect came firmly into the public domain in 1988, at a large conference in London organised by the British Geriatrics Society and Age Concern England. In one of the conference papers, Horrocks analysed twelve consecutive Health Advisory Service reports on long-stay wards in hospitals. Their findings of institutional abuse included:

- wards were too large, unhomely, open, and revealing few personal possessions;
- the atmosphere was custodial;
- overcrowding with beds too close together;
- furniture was 'dilapidated' with no carpeting;
- evidence of excessive restraint;
- lack of privacy;
- half the units inspected had no written protocols on continence;
- catering was poor with lack of choice;
- the last meal was at 5 p.m. to suit the institution;

- some units had discussed care plans but only one had been implemented;
- poor staffing ratios;
- lack of mental stimulation.

(cited in Tomlin 1989: 11–12)

Tomlin (1989) commented: 'These examples reflect passive abuse on a massive scale.'

Quality as a requirement

As we reflect on the existence of abuse in institutions, both individual and institutionalised abuse, we do well to recognise that abuse in continuing care facilities occurs as Bennett *et al.* have pointed out 'with almost monotonous regularity' (1997: 98). But we know how to recognise and even prevent most abuse in institutions. The answer is *quality* – well-trained staff, increased resources, a positive environment and user-friendly management systems, with proper complaints procedures and increased inspection and monitoring of establishments.

It is one thing to say this but the reality, as Nazarko has suggested, is that:

> Nursing homes are run as businesses with the aim of maximising profits by reducing costs. They are labour-intensive business and their greatest cost is staff wages, any nursing home proprietors seek to maximise profits by paying below the Whitley Council scales.
>
> (1995: 57)

Sexual abuse in residential settings

It would be irresponsible in this brief chapter to omit reference to the infrequently discussed subject of the sexual abuse of older persons, because this is as relevant an issue in residential settings as it is in domestic situations, and should not be ignored (Ramsey-Klawsnik 1991: 73–90; 1996: 67–87; Ker 1996: 166–71; Decalmer 1997: 41–74 *passim*).

Sexual abuse itself is identified less often than are other forms of elder mistreatment and the whole question of sexuality in later life is faced with what Ker has described as a 'double whammy taboo' (1996: 166). First, sexuality in older age is still not part of a general discourse about older people's self-value and their continuing involvement in life.

Second, the concept of the sexual abuse of old people is abhorrent to very many as being even a remote possibility. But sexual offenders are attracted by the vulnerability and availability of their potential victims and those who suffer from physical and mental impairment may be especially at risk. The sexual assault of elderly women and sometimes elderly men may be perpetrated by family members, caregivers and others who have regular access to elderly people, and who are often in positions of trust or authority. Because of this and because of the complexity of human relationships, the training of staff in the recognition and assessment of sexual abuse and in policies, procedures and intervention strategies is essential.

The lack of research

It is astonishing that with all the evidence that there is in the public domain, no British government has understood that there is a public responsibility and obligation to fund research that will enable us to understand better the issues that have been raised in this chapter. We need to understand why maltreatment of patients in residential settings occurs at all. We need to know much more about staff–patient conflict and the issues of restraint, over-medication, withholding of medication and under-nutrition within the context of long-term care. Furthermore, the political will to regulate and monitor all continuing care settings appears to be virtually absent (Bennett *et al.* 1997).

As Holstein has said:

> Practitioners rarely have the luxury of working in ideal circumstances. For those who work with abused and neglected older adults, the likelihood of achieving an ideal solution is slim. While the public may be appalled at newspaper descriptions of elder mistreatment, that dismay rarely translates into political action. Despite outrage, few understand the roots of problems that lead to elder abuse and neglect, and therefore few assume responsibility for activities designed to address these deeper causes. It is unlikely that this picture will change in the immediate future.
>
> (1996: 180)

Meanwhile, the size of the ageing population continues to increase with all that that implies for the future of long-term care.

References

Baillon, S., Boyle, A., Neville, P.G. and Scothern G. (1996) 'Factors that contribute to stress in care staff in nursing homes for the elderly', *International Journal of Geriatric Psychiatry* 11: 219–26.

Bennett, G.C.J. and Kingston, P. (1993) *Elder Abuse: Concepts, Theories and Interventions*, London: Chapman & Hall.

Bennett, G.C.J., Kingston, P. and Penhale, B. (1997) *The Dimensions of Elder Abuse: Perspectives for Practitioners*, Basingstoke: Macmillan.

CARIE (Coalition of Advocates for the Rights of the Infirm Elderly) (1991) *Ensuring an Abuse-Free Environment: A Learning Program for Nursing Home Staff*, Philadelphia: CARIE.

Clough, R. (1981) *Old Age Homes*, London: Allen & Unwin.

—— (1988a) *Scandals in Residential Centres: A Report to the Wagner Committee*, unpublished report.

—— (1988b) 'Danger: Look out for abuse', *Care Weekly*, 7 January.

—— (1996) 'The abuse of residents', in R. Clough (ed.) *The Abuse of Care in Residential Institutions*, London: Whiting & Birch.

—— (1999) 'Scandalous care: Interpreting public inquiry reports of scandals in residential care', *Journal of Elder Abuse and Neglect* 10(1/2) (in press).

Counsel and Care (1991) *Not Such Private Places*, London: Counsel and Care.

—— (1992) *What If They Hurt Themselves*, London: Counsel and Care.

—— (1995) *Care Betrayed*, London: Counsel and Care.

Decalmer, P. (1993) 'Clinical presentation', in P. Decalmer and F. Glendenning (eds) *The Mistreatment of Elderly People*, second edition, London: Sage.

—— (1997) 'Clinical presentation and management', in P. Decalmer and F. Glendenning (eds) *The Mistreatment of Elderly People*, second edition, London: Sage.

Doty, P. and Sullivan, E.W. (1983) 'Community involvement in combating abuse, neglect and maltreatment in nursing homes', *Milbank Fund Quarterly/Health and Society* 32: 222–51.

Eastley, R.J., Macpherson, R., Richards, H. and Mia, I.H. (1993) 'Assaults on professional carers of elderly people', *British Medical Journal* 307: 845.

Fader, A., Koge, N., Gupta, K.L. and Gambert, S.R. (1990) 'Perceptions of elder abuse by health care workers in a long-term care setting', *Clinical Gerontologist* 10(2): 87–9.

Ferguson, L. (1996) 'Bad apple or sick building?: Management responses to institutional abuse', in R. Clough (ed.) *The Abuse of Care in Residential Institutions*, London: Whiting & Birch.

Foner, N. (1994) 'Nursing home aides: Saints or monsters?', *The Gerontologist* 34(2): 245–50.

Glendenning, F. (1993) 'What is elder abuse and neglect?', in P. Decalmer and F. Glendenning (eds) *The Mistreatment of Elderly People*, London: Sage.

—— (1996) 'The mistreatment of elderly people in residential institutions', in R. Clough (ed.) *The Abuse of Care in Residential Institutions*, London: Whiting & Birch.

—— (1997) 'The mistreatment and neglect of elderly people in residential institutions: Research outcomes', in P. Decalmer and F. Glendenning (eds) *The Mistreatment of Elderly People*, second edition, London: Sage.

Glendenning, F. and Kingston, P. (eds) (1999) *Journal of Elder Abuse and Neglect* 10(1/2) (in press).

Goffman, E. (1968) *Asylums*, Harmondsworth: Penguin.

Goodridge, D.M., Johnston, P. and Thomson, M. (1996) 'Conflict and aggression in the work environment of nursing assistants: Implications for institutional elder abuse', *Journal of Elder Abuse and Neglect* 8(1): 49–68.

Halamandaris, V.J. (1983) 'Fraud and abuse in nursing homes', in J.I. Kosberg (ed.) *Abuse and Maltreatment of the Elderly: Causes and Interventions*, Boston: John Wright.

Harman, H. and Harman, S. (1989) *No Place Like Home: A Report of the First Ninety-Six Cases of the Registered Homes Tribunal*, London: NALGO.

Higgs, P. and Victor, C. (1993) 'Institutional care and the life course', in S. Arber and M. Evandrou (eds) *Ageing, Independence and the Life Course*, London: Jessica Kingsley.

Holmes, B. and Johnson, A. (1988) *Cold Comfort: The Scandal of Private Rest Homes*, London: Souvenir Press.

Holstein, M. (1996) 'Multidisciplinary decision-making: Uniting differing professional perspectives', in T.J. Johnson (ed.) *Elder Mistreatment: Ethical Issues, Dilemmas and Decisions*, New York: Haworth Press.

Howard, A. (1990) *Crossman: The Pursuit of Power*, London: Jonathan Cape.

Hughes, B. (1995) *Older People and Community Care: Critical Theory and Practice*, Buckingham: Open University Press.

Keller, B.H. (1996) 'A model abuse prevention training program for long-term care staff', in L.A. Baumhover and S.C. Beall (eds) *Abuse, Neglect and Exploitation of Older Persons: Strategies for Assessment and Intervention*, London: Jessica Kingsley.

Ker, H.J. (1996) 'Training residential staff to be aware of sexual abuse in old age', in R. Clough (ed.) *The Abuse of Care in Residential Institutions*, London: Whiting & Birch.

Kimsey, L.R., Tarbox, A.R. and Bragg, D.F. (1981) 'Abuse of the elderly, the hidden agenda: The caretakers and the categories of abuse', *American Geriatrics Society Journal* 22: 465–72.

Kosberg, J.I. (ed.) (1983) *Abuse and Maltreatment of the Elderly: Causes and Interventions*, Boston: John Wright.

Kosberg, J.I. and Garcia, J.L. (1995) *Elder Abuse: International and Cross-Cultural Perspectives*, New York: Haworth Press.

Lachs, M.S. and Pillemer, K.A. (1995) 'Abuse and neglect of elderly persons', *New England Journal of Medicine* 332(7): 437–43.

McCreadie, C. (1981) *Elder Abuse: An Exploratory Study*, London: Age Concern Institute of Gerontology, King's College London.

—— (1996) *Elder Abuse: Update on Research*, London: Age Concern Institute of Gerontology, King's College London.

Martin, J.P. (1984) *Hospitals in Trouble*, Oxford: Blackwell.

Maslach, C. (1982) *Burnout: The Cost of Caring*, Englewood Cliffs, NJ: Prentice-Hall.

Monk, A., Kay, L.W. and Litwin, H. (1984) *Resolving Grievances in Nursing Homes: A Study of the Ombudsman's Program*, New York: Columbia University Press.

Nazarko, L. (1996) 'The single care home', *Nursing Times* 92(4): 31–3.

Peace, S., Kellaher, L. and Willcocks, D. (1997) *Re-Evaluating Residential Care*, Buckingham: Open University Press.

Phillipson, C. and Biggs, S. (1992) *Understanding Elder Abuse: A Training Manual for Helping Professionals*, London: Longman.

—— (1995) 'Elder abuse: A critical overview', in P. Kingston and B. Penhale (eds) *Family Violence and the Caring Professions*, London: Macmillan.

Pillemer, K.A. (1988) 'Maltreatment of patients in nursing homes', *Journal of Health and Social Behaviour* 29(3): 227–38.

—— (1996) Private communication.

Pillemer, K.A. and Bachman-Prehn, R. (1991) 'Helping and hurting: Predictors of maltreatment of patients in nursing homes', *Research on Aging* 13(1): 74–95.

Pillemer, K.A. and Hudson, B. (1993) 'A model abuse prevention program for nursing assistants', *The Gerontologist* 33(1): 128–31.

Pillemer, K.A. and Moore, D.W. (1989) 'Abuse of patients in nursing homes: Findings from a survey of staff', *The Gerontologist* 29(3): 313–20.

—— (1990) 'Highlights from a study of abuse in nursing homes', *Journal of Elder Abuse and Neglect* 29(1/2): 5–19.

Ramsey-Klawsnik, H. (1991) 'Elder sexual abuse: Preliminary findings', *Journal of Elder Abuse and Neglect* 3(3): 73–90.

—— (1996) 'Assessing physical and sexual abuse in health care settings', in L.A. Baumhover and S.C. Beall (eds) *Abuse, Neglect and Exploitation of Older Persons: Strategies for Assessment and Intervention*, London: Jessica Kingsley.

Robb, B. (1967) *Sans Everything: A Case to Answer*, Edinburgh: Nelson.

Sinclair, I. (ed.) (1988) *Residential Care: The Research Reviewed*, vol. 2 of the Wagner Committee report, London: HMSO.

Solomon, K. (1983) 'Intervention for victimized elderly and sensitization of health professionals', in J.I. Kosberg (ed.) *Abuse and Maltreatment of the Elderly: Causes and Interventions*, Boston: John Wright.

Stannard, C. (1973) ' "Old folks and dirty work": The social conditions for patient abuse in a nursing home', *Social Problems* 20: 329–42.

Stathopoulos, P.A. (1983) 'Consumer advocacy and abuse of elders in nursing homes', in J.I. Kosberg (ed.) *Abuse and Maltreatment of the Elderly: Causes and Interventions*, Boston: John Wright.

Tarbox, A.R. (1983) 'The elderly in nursing homes: The psychological aspects of neglect', *Clinical Gerontologist* 1: 39–52.

Tomlin, S. (1989) *Abuse of Elderly People: An Unnecessary and Preventable Problem*, London: British Geriatrics Society.

Townsend, P. (1962) *The Last Refuge*, London: Routledge.

Townsend, P. and Davidson, N. (1982) *Inequalities in Health: The Black Report*, Harmondsworth: Penguin.

UKCC (United Kingdom Central Council for Nursing) (1994) *Professional Conduct Occasional Report on Standards of Nursing in Nursing Homes*, London: UKCC.

Vousden, M. (1987) 'Nye Bevan would turn in his grave', *Nursing Times* 83(32): 18–19.

Wagner Committee (1988) *Residential Care: A Positive Choice, Report of the Independent Review of Residential Care*, vol. 1, London: HMSO.

Wardhaugh, J. and Wilding, P. (1993) 'Towards an explanation of the corruption of care', *Critical Social Policy* 47: 4–31.

Wiener, C.L. and Kayser-Jones, J. (1990) 'The uneasy fate of nursing home residents: An organizational-interaction perspective', *Sociology of Health and Illness* 12(1): 84–104.

Willcocks, D., Pearce, S. and Kellaher, L. (1986) *Private Lives in Public Places*, London: Tavistock.

9 The abuse of older people in institutional settings

Residents' and carers' stories

Les Bright

> You just give up worrying about those sort of things, you have to accept that other people will be making all the important decisions for you now.

Counsel and Care provides information, advice and advocacy for older people and their carers on a wide range of matters connected with their welfare. The advice service is long-established and particularly well-known for the quality and depth of knowledge and experience about residential care and nursing homes. Alongside this direct work with individuals in need we have also been carrying out a programme of research examining the quality of care in homes for older people. Characteristically, the research consists of interviews with residents and staff that then go on to form the core of a publication intended to influence policy and practice. The publication is then used as a vehicle for organising mainly local conferences and training events, in partnership with other bodies such as inspection units, homes associations or groups of homes in the private, public or voluntary sectors. This programme of work has covered diverse topics: leisure and recreation, meals and mealtimes, healthcare, spiritual and personal values, and abuse.

Our work on abuse could not begin in the usual way, with interviews in homes, as we did not wish to create alarm and anxiety among the resident population, nor did we think that owners or managers would readily offer us access to their residents and staff group to discuss such a sensitive topic. Instead, we convened a series of seminars to which we invited a cross-section of the stakeholders to discuss their perceptions of the incidence and scope of abusive behaviour within homes. Publication of the report produced as a result of these consultations attracted a high level of media interest, with coverage on all the BBC television news bulletins on one day in late 1995, leading to many calls from members of the public anxious to tell stories, to seek information, reassurance or support for their 'campaigns' (Bright 1995). Most of the stories told here draw on the experiences related to me over the following months. All names have been changed to ensure confidentiality to those who told their story, joining with Counsel and Care to bring about changes in practices in care homes. The chapter also includes material drawn from the experience of delivering a training workshop on abuse with managers and staff of homes across the UK over the past two and a half years.

Alice was 100 years old, and had been resident in the same care home for more than ten years when I met her. She made the statement at the head of this chapter while I was sitting in her room for the second consecutive Friday afternoon. I had been engaged by the housing association that owned and managed her home to act as a source of independent advice and support for some of the residents of the home whom they thought might have been the subjects of wrong-doing by a former manager. All residents who might have been affected had been informed that I was around and could provide help if they felt they needed it. Alice was only one of two people who decided to take up the service. On the first occasion that I met her we had settled down in her room to talk about her concerns, when after only a short period of time the door was thrown open by a member of the care staff carrying towels, which she placed on the bed. She looked at us – and addressed me – 'Sorry, I didn't know you were here', and left the room, closing the door behind her. I wanted to discuss the issue of privacy with Alice but felt that this represented a hijacking by me of the agenda for our meeting. So, I said nothing. Our conversation carried on, but she was becoming tired and we decided that I should return the following week.

On the following Friday afternoon I returned, and we picked up the threads of our conversation. We had only been together for a very short time when the door was thrust open by the same member of staff as the previous week. Again, she was carrying towels, which she left on the bed. Once again, she made no communication with Alice, this time saying, 'Oh, it's you again.' This time I couldn't resist raising the matter with Alice, whose reply is quoted above.

Is such practice abusive? And, is it serious enough to warrant our concern? Is there anything we can do about it? There ought to be no hesitation in identifying such practice as abusive or in deciding that, in common with other daily practices that so diminish the often impover-ished life-styles of residents in care homes, we should be concerned and concerned enough to do something about it. But this professional response, that says that bad practice must be challenged regardless of the gravity of the particular action, runs counter to the view expressed by this resident, and perhaps many others too. She had adapted her life-style and expectations to fit with the reality of life in the institution in which she is looked after. She does not demand – nor expect to be given – either privacy or a say in the performance of the staff who look after her. She stopped short of repeating the words another resident in a different home uttered: 'My life is over now, I simply fit in with what I have been told I have to do.' Those words give life to theoretical propositions about abusive institutions that exist for the benefit of the people who work in them rather than the people who live in them. This is a theme I will return to later.

Degrading routine

Betty went to live in a nursing home because the social services care manager involved in assessing her needs determined that she was no longer capable of looking after herself at home, and was convinced that this would be the best option for her. Betty accepted this judgement, albeit reluctantly, and her small circle of friends felt a sense of relief that she would now get the kind of help she needed and which they were unable to give. Within a relatively short space of time Betty became unhappy and depressed. Whenever friends visited – and they did most days – she told them of the indignities she now experienced. Never before had she considered eating breakfast whilst emptying her bowels, but that became the norm with a care assistant who told her that she did not have enough time to get all the jobs done without adopting this time-saving routine, placing Betty on a bedpan while feeding her. When Betty resisted, the care assistant became yet more determined and handled her roughly, her actions accompanied by harsh words. Unhappiness and depression gave way to fear, itself accompanied by a decision to do or say nothing that would inflame the situation further. Betty followed Alice's advice to give up worrying, and to accept that other people will make all the decisions. Her friends were diplomatic but determined; they did nothing to inflame the situation but at the same time they pursued their concerns about the regime through the health authority's inspectorate, with the care manager, and the matron of the home, following information and advice from my agency. Just as Alice's expectations had changed over time so also had those of Betty's friends, to the extent that they needed reassurance that they were not making unrealistic and unachievable demands on the team providing care for Betty. Such an incident might be seen as an isolated example of an over-enthusiastic and undertrained care assistant; indeed, that is how it was for a time characterised by those with whom her friends raised the matter. Evidence from others' work tells us that such appalling practice is more widespread than any of us would prefer to believe. Patients 'were hauled out of bed ... plonked on commodes in their wet night clothes. Throned in indignity, this was where they had breakfast' (Jenkins 1997). Reveille at a nursing home in Britain, in the late 1990s – at 5.00 a.m. So, maybe Betty was telling the truth, and was not just trying to cause trouble for a member of staff against whom she had taken a dislike, as had been suggested by one of the professionals responding to the concerns her friends raised through the complaints system.

Wally's daughter visited him regularly. Most of the time his pleasure at seeing her was affected by the embarrassment he felt at being wet, and sometimes smelly too. His shame was matched by his daughter's distress at seeing her Dad in this way. She too had low expectations and asked us if there was anything she could do about the situation, or was being wet and dirty the price to be paid for being old and in need of care? We encouraged her to raise her concerns about the standard of care, and especially the continence management regime. Perhaps if Wally had remained independent in the community a feature of his life would have been persistent embarrassment and discomfort but the move to a home was intended to make life better in a number of ways. The care home manager listened sympathetically to the story and explained that the pressure to limit the number of pads per patient per day had come from her managers outside the home who were seeking economies in the face of increased costs. Though staff costs are a big proportion of the weekly expenses of any home it is not easy to reduce staffing levels without compromising the requirements of registration and risking a showdown with the inspectors. In such circumstances the search for economies can extend to incontinence pads, and savings may be found at the expense of residents. External pressure to reduce costs had an immediate impact on the quality of Wally's life, and that of his daughter too, but this need not have been the outcome if an individual toileting programme adjusted in the light of his needs, and the resources available to respond to them, had been the starting point for considering how to ensure that Wally's life still had some quality and that he was able to retain his dignity and face his daughter's visits with pleasure and pride.

Keeping up appearances

Bill's mother, Violet, had always taken pride in her appearance and so it came as a shock to him when over a period of months, coinciding with her move to residential care, she began to be less well groomed. Initially, her hair was not brushed, then her clothes looked grubby – and eventually shabby – with the final humiliation being to see her one day without her teeth, wearing a dress that didn't fit and that did not belong to her, and with only one stocking. Bill discussed the situation that had developed with his mother's key worker and another member of staff with whom Violet had established a warm rapport during her time at the home. They explained that new residents being admitted to the home were generally older, physically and mentally more frail and in need of significantly more help than envisaged within the statement of aims, the levels of staffing and the skill mix of the staff team. It was no longer possible to devote as much time to assisting Violet with her grooming or the selection of an appropriate outfit because staff were assisting doubly incontinent residents to the toilet, or were frequently at their wits' end trying to control aggressive residents with dementing illnesses. Staff suggested that such residents were in a residential care home because they could no longer manage independently, but the level of personal need was such that they should be allocated a place in a nursing home. Sadly, financial constraints meant that cheaper residential care won out over a provision more suited to these residents' care needs, but costing £100 per week more. As time went by, Bill realised that the level of staffing affected many other things including the level of supervision and the management of staff time, as well as staff's individual and collective demeanour. Staff became less interested and more introverted; standards fell and rules were introduced that had little or no connection to the provision of a quality service.

If these examples of falling standards, poor practice and lack of leadership are coupled with the growth in cases coming before the United Kingdom Central Council on Nursing, Midwifery and Health Visiting (UKCC) Professional Conduct Committee (Waters 1997), and the increasingly frequent reports in the trade press of cases coming before both Magistrates Courts and Crown Courts (to say nothing of the unrecorded summary dismissals of staff who fail to perform in a way that brings credit on the caring professions), then the case for a strengthened system of inspection, the establishment of a General Social Care Council, and a thorough and properly resourced awareness campaign becomes unanswerable. Taken along with the essential context of a largely untrained workforce who may do things, or fail to do things, because they know no better, our concern should be heightened even further.

Views from the field

Since the spring of 1996 I have travelled across the UK running a one-day workshop on the theme of abuse, designed specifically for people working with older people in residential care and nursing homes. At the time of writing, nearly 2,000 people working as carers and managers from the public, private and voluntary sectors have attended the workshop entitled 'Abuse, by any other name' (Bright 1997). The goals of the day are suitably modest:

- to raise awareness among those attending about the range of ways in which residents may be abused;
- to encourage them to share examples of good care practice;
- to empower participants to challenge bad practice and abusive behaviour.

Many of those attending arrive with a level of scepticism they reserve for trainers, writers, campaigners and others whom they consider poorly placed to comment on the difficulty of the job they undertake in looking after frail and vulnerable elderly people. But the tide turns fairly early on when they are asked to draw on *their* practice knowledge to develop their own thinking about abuse. Action on Elder Abuse's (AEA) thirty-three-word, carefully constructed definition is deconstructed in order that each part – and the interdependency of the parts – can be understood:

> Elder abuse is a single or repeated act or lack of appropriate action occurring within any relationship where there is an expectation of trust, which causes harm or distress to an older person.
>
> (AEA 1995)

This definition presents a problem because even people who are interested in the topic find it difficult to memorise such a lengthy statement, and those who may not be wholly convinced that there is a problem will find it much more difficult to do so. In any event, such a definition does not easily connect with the experience of their daily routines and tasks. Discussion of the commonly accepted types of abuse: physical, psychological, financial, sexual and neglect brings the topic closer to that experience, yet it is still much too easy to respond with the tired phrase: 'It couldn't happen here.' After all, most of the time most older residents are not being physically assaulted by care staff, are not having their money or possessions stolen, and are not suffering sexual assaults. However, it seems that far too many of them are subjected to psychological abuse in the form of name-calling, being ignored or being spoken to unpleasantly, and a significant number of residents will experience neglect in one or more of the ways in which it can surface: being made to wait too long for the toilet, not receiving attention for a physical or mental health need soon enough, or being fed a poor diet with little food that they enjoy (Bright 1997). Recent research, conducted on behalf of the Office of Fair Trading (1998) as part of its inquiry into consumer issues in residential care, reveals that the three concerns most often mentioned by the 965 people whom they interviewed were (in no particular order) inexperienced staff, deteriorating standards and too little food. They also said that staff had too little time to talk to them. There is a strong link between these findings, arising from a Government-sponsored inquiry, and the kinds of practices described by care staff working in homes.

Course participants are asked to consider the question, 'What do you see, experience or even participate in that gives you cause for concern about the way in which older people are looked after?' Working in small groups, to encourage discussion, they are asked to write their thoughts on cards that they will look at later with a view to forming an opinion on the seriousness of each of the statements they and their colleagues have made. Statements such as shouting at people, and hitting people, are given as examples of the kinds of things people might write on their cards. In a very short space of time a large amount of material is generated. Some words figure many times over: 'ignoring them', 'talking about them as if they are not there', 'making people wait', 'denying choice', and 'affronts to dignity' appear so many times that it would be possible for an outsider to form the view that it is normal to ignore people, to discuss them and their most intimate needs in front of them without their involvement, to make people wait so long for the toilet that it is too late by the time that they are taken there and to remove resident choice about everything from when they get up to what they eat, or do with their time. However, many workshops tend to throw up words and deeds that have not figured in previous discussions. So, alongside the statements to which I have become inured over time, are added bizarre activities undertaken – repeatedly or on a one-off basis – by care staff in the course of looking after people.

In writing a policy on how to look after people in a residential care or nursing home it would not have occurred to me to tell staff that they should not listen in, on the intercom system, to resident conversations in their rooms as a form of staff entertainment. It was only after a care assistant had written this down, as a concern she had about life at the home she worked in, that I realised that it was necessary to start a long way back in the process of identifying how residents are subjected to a dripping tap of indignities. Only after appreciating that such activities arise daily, and are not commented on, can steps be taken to turn things around. 'Spitting' has appeared on the cards on a couple of occasions, demonstrating that some staff respond to the older people in their care in the way that they might have done in the past with their own children; as one participant explained the situation: 'When my son pulled another boy's hair I pulled his so that he understood how painful it was, and when he started spitting I spat at him too – he soon learned not to do it.'

Staff spit at residents because residents spit at them! The same explanation is used to justify staff striking out at residents: 'Lots of them aren't angels, you know; we put up with a lot, they try to touch you up and some of the men are still very strong. It's the only thing they understand.' While it may be true that some residents are still quite physically strong, and in line with their behaviour throughout life they express themselves physically by pushing and shoving, or forcing their attentions on other people, that cannot be any more than a superficial explanation for how some staff respond to the threat. In too many cases staff use such an analysis as a justification for falling below acceptable standards of behaviour for a staff member. As the population of care homes becomes older on admission and more mentally frail (Moniz-Cook *et al.* 1998), the task confronting care staff becomes even more demanding, leading to many situations in which those who believe that the older person will only learn from experience exact humiliating revenge by inhuman acts.

Asked to look dispassionately at the cards, produced anonymously by other participants, most find it easy enough to identify unacceptable behaviours. Many of these statements promote discussion, particularly those which identify the many ways in which residents' needs are subjugated to routine and are excluded from decisions about daily life. It was the enduring pattern of ensuring that residents were all out of bed and dressed by an agreed time that led Betty being fed her meal while sitting on a bedpan. If staff had cared about Bill's mother as someone who deserved their attention, to maintain her once proud appearance, would they have allowed her to appear so dishevelled? And wouldn't the 'towel-lady' have spoken to Alice, rather than me, when she came into the room during our confidential discussion if she had respect for Alice's privacy?

The picture that emerges is of routines that become established and are maintained without any reference to the principles and values commonly accepted as fundamental to providing a good quality of life and good-quality care. Those who seek to protect and promote the welfare of older people living in homes need to address resource issues in the context of valuing older people. Routines need to benefit the resident group rather than the demands of the rota (Bright 1999).

Families' perspectives

So far I have chosen to direct attention towards matters of detail, largely because they reflect the range of problems that I have confronted in advising older people and, more often, their relatives, or because they are topics that arise from contact with people working at all levels in the field. There are, however, other cases that serve to remind us that, contrary to the belief that we would wish to hold, some homes fail to provide the safety and security residents and their families are seeking in making the decision to move into a home.

David was one of the people who contacted Counsel and Care after the television coverage of our campaign to highlight abuse in care homes, telling me the sad story of his mother, Meg. Meg entered a home at the age of 87 because David and his family became increasingly concerned about her safety, as she had started to wander the streets late at night, as a consequence of the onset of dementia, to be returned home to her flat in a police car. When they requested help from social services they were impressed with the speed, skill and resourcefulness of the assessment, and the way in which plans were made, taking care to leave the family with the final choice about whether or not it would be possible to support her at home. David was himself nearly of pensionable age and had suffered a major scare with a heart attack, and so reluctantly it was decided that his mother should be found a place in a nursing home. Meg settled in to her new home fairly quickly and David or another family member visited almost every day. Over the next six months she was the victim of three unexplained incidents. On the first occasion she was admitted to hospital with a broken wrist. Her family was understanding and in no way condemning of the staff of the home, recognising that this increasingly frail old lady was as likely to fall in her new home as in the flat she had left behind. They did expect, however, that the home's manager or another staff member would be able to tell them where or when the incident had occurred, and were disappointed to learn that the home had absolutely no idea. Their disappointment turned to anger when they discovered another unexplained injury when they visited her in her hospital bed. Staff were as puzzled about this as they had been about the original 'accident'. The accident book provided no clues, and the key worker who had responsibility for Meg did not recall ever having seen the injury.

David and his daughter continued to visit Meg and, looking back, sensed changes. Ownership had passed to another company and operational management changed too, with a new manager coming in to replace the matron with whom the family felt they had established a rapport. The client group being looked after also seemed to change, with more mentally ill people, some of whom were significantly younger than Meg, being accommodated. Shortly after this, Meg's wedding ring disappeared. She had not been without it since she married her late husband more than sixty years before and she became very distressed and agitated. The family were initially told that the home was not insured against such eventualities and staff seemed uninterested in either their resident's distress or the family's indignation. The management relented and made a payment to purchase a replacement ring, but by then the damage had been done, and clearly Meg remained upset. While it might have been the case that Meg had misplaced it herself and in her confused state had been unable to locate it, that was not the view which the family formed. Their misgivings reached a new level when David received a telephone call alerting him to the hospitalisation of his mother with 'a superficial injury to the face'. When he and his daughter arrived at the hospital they found Meg lying in bed in a confused and distressed state with a severely swollen, discoloured and lacerated face. Once again, nobody at the home was able to provide an explanation as to how she had received the injury, in the middle of the night. She was by then so frail as to be unable to get out of bed unassisted, and could not walk at all. On her return to the home, plans were made, with the help of the original care manager from social services, to move Meg to another home in the locality. Within five weeks Meg had died, but David's and his family's distress lingered on. They blamed themselves for not having reacted sooner to the feelings that they now so clearly held about the home, and for not having been more persistent in their questioning of key staff members and the home's inspectorate. They do not know whether Meg had been struck once, or more than once, by another resident with dementia, or by a cruel staff member. Neither do they know whether there was a thief among the staff group, or simply too little supervision of residents and staff. They take the view that any of these would have detrimental effects on the welfare of the residents. And that is a view shared by professionals, not that the possibilities are interchangeable but that ultimately the effect on residents could be the same. Meg's safety had been a key factor in influencing the family to choose a home for her, but they found themselves wishing that they had somehow been able to find the resources to sustain her at home rather than to expose her to the dangers she experienced during those last few months of her life.

Dorothy was the victim of two serious sexual assaults by another resident at the local authority home where she lived. Her two daughters, who each lived at a considerable distance from the home, assumed that Dorothy would be well cared for and safe. They also expected to be told of any changes in her condition. These hopes went unmet with Dorothy being assaulted but no record being kept of this, nor any mention made to her daughters until a further assault, by the same man, led to the manager contacting one of them and asking her to visit on the morning following the second incident. It was only when this second assault was being described that the story of the previous incident, just two days earlier, which had caused great harm and distress to a very frail elderly lady, began to emerge. This event also exposed weaknesses in the procedures, awareness, and understanding of staff and managers who contacted neither Dorothy's family, nor the police, and failed to record the occurrence either at the time or in the course of the following few days. The first incident had involved a serious sexual assault, the extent of which was never fully established, where a male resident was found naked in bed with Dorothy demanding that she touch him intimately. He was removed to his own nearby room, under protest, and Dorothy was visited an hour later to check if she was alright. In the absence of evident deep distress, staff were simply told to keep an eye on her, and to carry on as normal, including offering her a bath, as the incident had taken place on the day when she would normally receive a bath. In the interest of maintaining normality, for what could be considered well-meaning reasons, any chance of forensic evidence to confirm the scenes witnessed by night care staff was washed away, literally. Events over the next few days did nothing to protect the resident who had been put at risk, nor to prevent a recurrence, as the dreadful follow-up revealed when the same man again visited Dorothy, on this occasion nearly suffocating her in addition to attempting intercourse.

What followed demonstrates the need for staff to be given clear guidance on dealing with such a situation, precisely because it is so unusual and potentially very damaging for the individual and her immediate family. There appeared to be no policy for dealing with such an incident, no procedures to be followed by staff, and no guidelines for those who might be confronted with such a difficult situation. As management and staff wrestled with the professional dilemmas that seemed to have surrounded them, they exhibited a lack of clarity about their primary task of protecting and promoting the welfare of residents, and a sad lack of insight into the impact of such incidents on others. They seemed to believe that if they kept quiet about it the problem would – like the perpetrator, a user of the respite service – just go away, at least in the short term. As senior managers tried to explain away the problem by reference to the complex demands of a more dependent group of residents, it became clear that the staff were expected to provide a planned and sensitive service without having sufficient and appropriate information about people admitted to the home for respite. Care plans, where they existed, simply prescribed the need for respite, without describing the characteristics of the individual and the resources needed to ensure that, in providing a family with respite, they were not inflicting a major problem on the community the respite user would be joining. In this case the respite user's behaviour was not so challenging as to be outside the competence of the staff working at the home, it was just not communicated before his arrival, nor raised by staff after they had removed him from the room he entered uninvited to commit the first assault.

Inaction by staff may be attributable to weaknesses in responding to male sexuality, or in identifying the possibility that he might behave in ways for which he could not be held responsible, and for which they must make preparations to prevent damage to others. As has been the experience in many other cases where a resident's relatives have complained about the care being provided, the complaints process itself becomes hurtful. Staff have not always distinguished themselves by providing full, clear and honest accounts of the events, and their own or colleagues' part in them, and the level of confidence that relatives then display has been affected as a consequence. This lack of confidence may be expressed openly or implied and has the effect of driving a wedge between families and staff to whom they have entrusted the care of a relative. However, the business of investigating a complaint may also have the effect of identifying other shortcomings in the management, supervision and organisation of the home. A process originating in a real concern about one person's care has the potential to develop a broader and positive focus whereby deep-seated poor practice may be exposed to view for the first time.

Conclusion

If we consider Alice's lack of privacy as being important and worthy of attention to the same degree as Dorothy's fate at the hands of another resident, or Violet's decline in appearance as worrying as Betty breakfasting on the bedpan, the messages are quite clear: the quality of care in homes can be affected in many different ways and, regardless of the severity, it is possible to challenge and change these practices. Vulnerable residents, however, may be reluctant or unable to speak out.

Privacy rather than isolation can, and must, be established and maintained, and the power to do that lies in the hands of managers and staff. Telling staff what is necessary to achieve acceptable levels of privacy is a relatively simple task, but monitoring how those instructions are followed will require determined work by managers – at least in the short term.

A desire for a safe and secure environment motivates many older people and their families to seek residential care (Department of Health 1994) and homes cannot afford to compromise on this issue. Attending to this goal simply by reference to the built environment ignores the importance of protecting residents from physical assault or sexual menaces. Safety can only be assured if staff are confident that they have full information at the time of admission and add to it with their own observations of residents' behaviour.

Protecting residents' dignity requires attention in many different directions to both the routines of the home and the ways in which they can de-personalise staff and residents, as well as respecting the individuality of the people being looked after. Degrading practices such as feeding while toileting diminish staff and residents alike and must not be tolerated. Dealing with such practice presents no difficulty at all: staff must be told that such behaviour is gross misconduct and leads to instant dismissal. There are no excuses for such appalling lapses.

Above all, we must create a climate in which staff are able to share their concerns about their own or colleagues' performance, and can receive honest feedback on the way in which they carry out their duties: let's praise good work, as a matter of routine, and condemn poor practice wherever it rears its head. The alternative is to hear continual stories from residents and their relatives of the very worst 'care'.

References

Action on Elder Abuse (1995) *Elder Abuse Information Leaflet*, London: Action on Elder Abuse.

Bright, L. (1995) *Care Betrayed*, London: Counsel and Care.

—— (1997) *Harm's Way*, London Counsel and Care.

—— (1999) 'Elder Abuse in Care and Nursing Settings Detection and Prevention' in P. Slater and M. Eastman (eds) *Elder Abuse: Critical Issues in Policy and Practice*, London: Age Concern England.

Department of Health (1994) *The F Factor*, Social Services Inspectorate, Department of Health, London: HMSO.

Jenkins, D. (1997) 'From hell hole to heaven', *Nursing Times* 93 (33) 27–9.

Moniz-Cook, E., Agar, S., Silver, M., Woods, R., Wang, M., Elston, C., *et al.* (1998) 'Can staff training reduce behavioural problems in residential care for the elderly mentally ill?', *International Journal of Geriatric Psychiatry* 13: 149–58.

Office of Fair Trading (1998) *Older People as Consumers in Care Homes*, London: Office of Fair Trading.

Waters, J. (1997) 'UKCC toughens up its act on conduct committee', *Nursing Times* 24(93): 6.

10 The abuse of older people in institutional settings

The role of management and regulation

Roger Clough

The statement that older people sometimes are abused in the places in which staff are expected to provide care needs frequent repetition. So, too, does the fact that what is termed 'abuse' is the assault, rape, or neglect of residents, or theft from them. Abuse in residential and nursing homes is particularly ugly and unpalatable because of the fact that people, in moving to a home, expect to be cared for. For harm to come from the staff in whom residents and relatives have placed trust is a frightening betrayal. That is not to claim that abuse is perpetrated only by staff: some abuse is perpetrated by residents.

Establishments designated as 'residential care homes' or 'nursing homes' are subject to regulation. This means that they have to be registered before they are allowed to function and are then inspected on a regular basis. The system current at the time of writing (1998) is that which follows the implementation of the NHS and Community Care Act, 1990, with amendments. Residential care homes are regulated by local authorities, typically based in social services departments though subject to oversight by the Chief Executive of the authority; by contrast, health authorities regulate nursing homes. There have been attempts by individual registration authorities to set the guidelines for registration, the procedures for inspection and procedures for making complaints (see Clough 1994: 1–26). More recently, energy has been expended in trying to ensure that residents, people representing residents and voluntary bodies participate in inspections.

This system has been criticised on two main grounds: first, the divide between residential care homes and nursing homes is artificial; and, second, local authorities have conflicts of interest in regulating local-authority homes as well as private and voluntary homes. The Government is to introduce new, regional structures for regulation based outside local authorities, with responsibility across the residential/nursing divide and, indeed, for domiciliary care. There may well be statements of 'required standards' to be met by all providers.

Imagine being in the position of a manager or an inspector at the time a report of abuse in another establishment is published. No doubt there will be competing feelings: repulsion at the events; relief that it did not take place in 'your' home; determination that such events never will happen there; fear that you can never be sure that something is not going badly wrong in some part of the home, at some time and between some people. It is no wonder that some agencies do not want to run residential homes, whether for children or adults; the task and responsibility appear too great.

What compounds the anxieties of management is the well-documented knowledge that the style of leadership and management makes a dramatic impact on the life of the home. There is considerable potential to influence the lives of residents. There is also the accompanying responsibility for what happens.

Constructing concepts of good and bad practice

The word *abuse* is vague until linked with other words in phrases such as 'abuse of power'. If we take the general usage in social care, we recognise that the term is used to describe practice that is improper and unacceptable from one person to another, who is a recipient of social-care services. The word on its own tells us nothing about the nature of the event, nor its severity. Often, the word is used loosely in phrases such as 'people being at risk of abuse'. Without further specification such phrases are meaningless, unless they recognise that everyone is at risk of abuse. We do know, though, that 'abuse' is used to refer to a position in which one person exerts power improperly over another.

The most usual examples of abuse quoted are of staff abusing residents. This must not blind us to the fact that residents sometimes abuse other residents and sometimes abuse staff, as Hilary Brown observes in Chapter 4. The construction of what is abuse must not avoid the uncomfortable reality that sometimes the people who abuse their power are residents.

I return to the generality of defining what is and is not acceptable. A relative of a resident or a new worker may see something about which they are concerned. They have limited knowledge and experience against which to test their concern. How should they view what they have seen? What should they do? Was the way in which a resident was held or manoeuvred by a member of staff acceptable?

One of the first essentials for management is that there is clarity about the objectives of the home, its systems and its practice. If people are to make judgements about what happens, they must know what is supposed to be happening and how the place is meant to work. Bad or unacceptable practice has to be defined against good or acceptable practice. This does not mean that the managers on their own undertake this task: their responsibility should be to involve all stakeholders in the construction of the statement of purpose. Defining good and bad practice should be in the context of that negotiation about task and purpose.

Further, there has often been an assumption that it is not necessary to define either good or bad practice on the assumption that people will recognise what it is. Yet, in residential childcare there are numerous examples of young people stating to inquiries that they had not complained about assaults because they had not known that it was not a part of what they should expect (Clough 1988).

There are now requirements that agencies running homes should inform residents about the procedures for making complaints. The information may be imparted in different ways, such as a part of individual leaflets to each resident or in general notices displayed on walls. People need to know *what* they may complain about and *how* to complain. However, given the dependence of residents on staff for the provision of services, commenting on perceived shortcomings will never be easy (see Chapter 5).

The construction of abuse may be undertaken as a discrete exercise in which lists of unacceptable behaviour from one person to another are defined: residents may not be ... slapped, punched and so on. Indeed, also, residents may not commit such acts against others. In constructing lists like this there is a tendency to move from gross behaviour such as hitting to activities that are more difficult to define, such as inappropriate touching or holding. There are dangers in such constructions in that they attempt to define what is unacceptable. What is unacceptable makes sense only in the context of what is acceptable. All the interested parties – residents, relatives, community, managers, regulators – should be involved in defining such terms so that all understand the implications of the statements produced. The best way forward may be for the Government to require the production of locally negotiated statements.

The purpose of considering good and bad practice is that these different groups of people should be clear about what is unacceptable practice. Whatever the reasons for unacceptable practice, its existence must be recognised and condemned. It is essential that this idea of *unacceptable practice* is established. This allows differentiation between a notion of *not good enough practice* (for example, 'I wish I had more time to spend with residents') and *unacceptable practice*. The purpose of this distinction is to focus first on describing and examining what has happened. As has been discussed already, people may not be certain as to the category that best describes an event they have seen. The test for all parties is to reach a conclusion on acceptability/unacceptability.

Let us consider a number of examples of life in a residential home for older people:

- a resident is hit by another person (staff or resident);
- a resident is held by someone and not allowed to do whatever she/he wanted;
- a staff member speaks harshly to a resident (threatening, bullying, belittling);
- a resident is thought not to be eating enough;
- a resident is wearing dirty clothes and smells unpleasant;
- a resident has a sexual relationship with another resident or staff member;
- a resident has less money than relatives expect.

Of course, the range of examples could be expanded. The purpose of listing the situations above is to develop ways to examine different types of event.

Some are unacceptable *in any circumstances*, and any form of hitting is one such. Others *nearly always* are unacceptable, illustrated by speaking harshly. There is need here for further definition of what and how things were said. The test is that it is reasonable on certain occasions for staff to speak firmly to residents but, whatever the provocation, staff should never intimidate, bully or demean residents.

All the other examples *may or may not* be unacceptable; the circumstances need to be examined. When a resident is not eating enough, the explanation may lie in the inadequacy of the food supplied (not enough food, not nutritious, poorly cooked or presented, unacceptable in terms of diet, too little choice) *or* in the condition or attitude of the resident. He/she may be ill and not want food, may have lost interest in living, be suffering from the effects of medication or may demand types of food that are beyond what can be provided in the home; in the last example, it is necessary to see what were the terms on which the resident moved into the home.

The resident who wears dirty clothes is likely to be an indicator of unacceptable care by the staff. Except in the very short term, it is possible for residents themselves and their clothes to be washed frequently enough to avoid dirt and smells. However, there may be a resident who refuses to wash and change clothes.

Sexual activity involves different types of test. The core test is whether both parties have consented, which in turn demands consideration of the competence of a person to consent. I would argue that although sexual relationships between staff and residents might be consensual, they should be regarded as unacceptable because of the power inherent in the staff position.

Judging relationships between residents has other complexities. First, residents, nearly always men, may sexually assault others. Staff at times are torn between wanting to allow people a sexual life, their attitudes differing towards sexuality of men and women, and the difficulties in determining whether or not someone is participating willingly. Consideration of competence is essential and people who are judged not to be competent to make such decisions must be protected.

The final example above refers to money. This one shows the necessity to take account of the interests of different parties. Relatives may be right in a claim that a resident's money is being stolen by another resident or staff. However, it may be that the resident is spending the money as she/he wishes, which may not be what the relatives want.

Thus, what has to be determined is the acceptability or unacceptability of practice. Whether the term 'abuse' is helpful or not in such discussions is debatable. Typically, 'abuse' is used to refer to one person with power over another abusing that power to the detriment of the other. Most of the situations above would fall into that category.

The reality of residential work

Frequently, there has been too little consideration of the reality of the task in residential care. Thus, the response to reports of staff assaults on residents sometimes involves agencies defining more and more precisely what staff may do, perhaps detailing where and how they may touch residents. The problem with such attempts to rule out abuse is that they are likely to distort daily living.

Residential work with older people requires intimate physical care of one person by another. Definitions to ensure that inappropriate physical contact is ruled out run the risk of creating sterile care in intimate situations, itself potentially abusive. The problem is that in the best practice people negotiate as to what they want from the other and have their wishes respected. The danger in allowing negotiation is that the wishes may not be respected. The starting point in constructing notions of good and bad practice is that residents *live* in the home and should have a say in how their care is organised. Without that, there is no human contact between people. Narrow, restrictive definitions of the task may stop good practice as well as bad: they may prevent a resident or staff member holding the other as a comfort when the person is upset.

Indeed, residential work, concerned as it is with the arrangements for living, creates dilemmas and pressures for residents and staff. One resident annoys another: whose responsibility is it to take action? A resident repeatedly walks outside the home and is thought by some people to be a risk to herself: what is to happen? Add further details to the example, perhaps that the resident often is confused and cannot remember where she was meant to be or from where she had come. Should staff find ways to stop her leaving the home? (Is this legal? Is it practical?) Living with other people and providing care and housing for other people produce responsibilities.

Take the mundane example of bathing: if a resident is insistent that she wants to bath on her own and recognises the risks involved, should she be allowed to do so? Who will be held to account if the resident has an accident?

There is a temptation in residential work to push the complexity away, to fail to acknowledge the tensions. In these circumstances everybody operates as if the competing demands of various people can be satisfied: the relative wanting to feel that her mother is safe; the resident wanting to take decisions for herself; the care assistant anxious that she cannot give as much time to help a particular person as she would want. Failing to acknowledge and work at the problems creates a veneer to practice under which the reality exists, a potentially dangerous state.

Management has to create the forum in which people can recognise the complexity of the task, define the purpose and be free to air their concerns.

The primary task

The Department of Health and Social Security (1973) sets out a general statement on the function of a home: 'The function of a home is to provide considerate and skilful care in comfortable surroundings for elderly people who, even with help, are unable to live in homes of their own' (p. 1) Individual agencies may add their own requirements. For example, Cumbria Social Services Inspectorate (CSSI) adds that all homes for adults '*must* produce clear statements which outline their policy, and these should be sufficiently detailed for residents and others to know the sort of home into which they are considering moving' (Clough 1994).

Clarity of purpose is regarded as one of the basic components of good practice:

> if a home is to run well everybody must know what it aims to do. There are many occasions when there are competing demands, in particular on staff, and it is the statement of purpose which should provide a ray of light. Of course without clarity of purpose it is impossible to evaluate the care provided. It is also vital to remember the ease with which a statement of purpose can be put aside. Like many other mission statements it can decorate the foyer without being related to practice.
>
> (Clough 1999b)

A recent publication on management suggests that people should:

> look at key documents such as the Home's philosophy or value statement, statement of aims and objectives, policies and procedures. Consider the values represented there.
>
> (Residential Forum 1997: 10)

It asks if people 'have or have adopted' the following: a 'mission statement; statement of aims and philosophy; equal opportunities policy; code of practice; health and safety policy; charter of service users' rights; complaints policy and procedures; recognised quality assurance or quality management systems' (1997: 10).

Burton argues that 'clarifying the primary task is the first act of management at every level'.

> The manager must ask herself or himself, 'What is this organisation here to do, and what is my part in it?' If the task is unclear, or if the task is found to be different at different levels or in different departments of the organisation, the service will deteriorate and the client will suffer.
>
> (1998: 48)

Thus, the reason why there is to be a statement of purpose is to ensure that everybody understands what the organisation exists to do. Good practice – and therefore bad practice – can only be understood if management has ensured that the primary task is defined. Following on from the construction of the primary task, there needs to be 'agreement with stakeholders as to objectives, values, methods and style' (Clough 1999b).

Building in quality

The emphasis in general management theory over the last twenty years has been on trying to ensure that the output is satisfactory first time around. The move has been from a focus on inspection at the end of a production line to weed out the faulty product, to ensuring that faulty products are not produced. Phrases like 'quality assurance' or 'building in quality' are attempts at creating systems in which the quality is assured during production. Different authors will stress different approaches and, of course, these will vary with the nature of the activity. Frequently mentioned factors are:

- clarity as to both task and systems: stress is placed on the need for all stakeholders to be involved in defining these activities; the temptation for managers is to define task and systems but this does not ensure the commitment of staff to the goals;
- the commitment of staff: the idea is that staff should internalise the ends of the organisation so that they have a commitment to maintaining the quality;
- supervision of staff: the chance for staff to review their practice and for managers to oversee their work;
- managers involved in some way in day-to-day activities so that they have direct experience of what is happening: they see, hear and smell the life of the home *and* they see how residents are feeling and behaving;
- the creation of an environment in which staff can give of their best: this will involve both working to agreed ends but also interpreting what to do when 'the rule book' does not provide the answer; sometimes this is listed as an opportunity for staff to be creative;
- systems for review of what happens: in residential work it is recognised that residents who are dependent on staff for care may be reluctant to criticise; various strategies are developed to encourage resident discussion of what goes on and for others, who may put forward the interests of residents, to do so on their behalf;
- a capacity to correct faults: too often organisations review their activities but fail to act on information;

- procedures for anyone to report their concerns about serious shortcomings in practice: these take many different forms and should be designed to make it easy for people to report; in addition, they may try to create a culture in which there is recognition that the prime loyalty of staff is to the primary task, in some way the care of residents; in other words, they are to be given a responsibility to express anxieties about the work of colleagues and should not evade this under mistaken notions of loyalty to colleagues or that it is not their business; the motto in this context is that 'bad practice is everybody's business'.

Quality assurance literature stresses 'customer focus'. There is abundant evidence that good residential practice must be *resident-centred*, and that is constructed to meet the needs and interests of individual residents (King *et al.* 1971; Parker 1988; Clough 1999b). As Bright identifies (in Chapter 9 of this volume) the focus must not be allowed to shift to one of being *institution-centred*, in which the end becomes that of 'doing the tasks' without recognising what the tasks were designed to achieve. In this distorted picture the end becomes 'getting residents up' or 'serving thirty meals' rather than negotiating with residents as to how they want to get up in the morning or how they like their meals.

The Residential Forum recognises that there are different 'customers': there are the residents but there are also the people who are purchasing care.

> Customer focus in this context has two aspects. One is to involve service users, relatives, their representatives and other stake holders in the Home to *develop* services tailored to their needs. The other is to use processes to assure that needs are met.
>
> (1997: 89–90)

Following this, the Residential Forum continues, managers should 'find out how satisfied customers are with the services they receive' (1997: 90).

The emphasis on assuring quality, in effect developing systems that will produce the desired end result, may lead to a concentration on the system rather than the product. Indeed, one position taken by proponents of quality assurance systems is that external managers and regulators should look at the quality assurance systems, but do not have to examine the end results. The basis of the argument is that if good enough systems are in place, the practice will itself be good enough. This is a dangerous argument, in particular as it is possible for a quality assurance system to focus on inessentials or on the way that practice is presented. My comment is not an attack on quality assurance, but a recognition of the limits of what it should be expected to achieve. Certainly, in a former job as a regulator, I would not have restricted regulation to inspection of quality assurance systems. Both managers and regulators must examine day-to-day life in the home.

The definition of abuse: whose problem?

The neat and short answer is 'everybody's'. It is common for different groups of people to have varying expectations of what should happen in a residential home. Determining what is unacceptable demands that there is as much agreement as possible as to the meaning of the terms. Take an obvious example of a resident who wants to go out of the home: staff may be anxious about the person's capacity or health; relatives may want the older person to be safe and put pressure on staff; regulators may have guidance on the circumstances in which residents may be stopped from leaving or the arrangements for when they want to go out. Alongside these views, there is the fact that residents are resident voluntarily and may not be detained against their will. In this cluster of competing interests what is to happen? Are staff in the home neglectful if they allow someone to leave when she/he wants or are they guilty of illegal containment if they prevent someone from leaving?

The importance of the example is that there is no neat, single answer. Homes have a responsibility to provide care, a part of which is protection and a part of which is the creation of an environment where people may live as they wish.

Learning from what goes wrong

In endeavouring to assure quality, the best management and regulation should take account of what we know about abuse in residential care and nursing homes. It is not safe for managers or regulators, in the belief that their own systems are satisfactory, to ignore what is known about the situations when abuse has taken place.

Causation of abuse

It is essential that managers and regulators are alert to the fact that abuse does not arise from a single cause; there is a temptation to focus on particular types of abuse or particular causes of abuse that have an impact on the individuals examining abusive situations. Such a mistaken analysis will ignore potential abuse on a wide front. Glendenning (in Chapter 8 of this volume) has reviewed the international evidence on the causation of abuse.

Building on an analysis by Rowlings (1995), I have argued elsewhere (Clough 1996: 6 and 1999a) that abuse is caused through an interplay between *structural* and *environmental* factors interacting with the *individual characteristics* of staff and residents and the *work style* of the staff group.

The *structural* category recognises the societal processes that structure perceptions of older people and the resources provided. Older people's interests are seen as less important than those of younger adults. Similarly, the task of tending others, that is providing for their physical well-being while taking account of their emotional needs, holds low status.

As well as this, people live and work in *environments* that may create stresses. Here there are elements related to the nature of the work and those related to resources: numbers and capabilities of staff, the way they are managed, and the conditions in which people live and work. In terms of the third category, *individual characteristics*, some people, staff or residents are more likely to abuse than others, although anybody under pressure has the potential to abuse. It is also becoming recognised that some people are more likely to be abused than others. This is not surprising. It is accepted that bullies bully particular types of people and abuse has similarities with such abuse of power. The final category stresses the importance of the way in which the staff team respond; people are influenced by environment and resources but have the potential to respond in different ways. The category *work style* refers to the ways in which staff work and the decisions made by them about practice. It recognises that staff have some ability to determine their approach to work.

As has been stated earlier, management has the responsibility to create the conditions in which the primary task of the home can be accomplished. In the same way, management should aim to counter the factors noted above which contribute to abuse. Thus, *in relation to structures*, management should aim to create a climate in which older people's views are taken seriously and any belittling is challenged. The need for such a climate emerges clearly from Les Bright's chapter in this volume, and is of particular importance for residents who most often have their views dismissed, for example people with dementia. Goldsmith stresses that 'it clearly is possible ... to hear the voice of people with dementia ... on a scale which is far beyond that which prevails today in most areas of service provision' (1997: 118). Another example of action on structures is to ensure that the contracts with individual residents are detailed, clearly written and specify what residents should do if they want to discuss their care.

In relation to environment, management has a responsibility to create a setting in which people can live and work well: appropriate buildings, plant and facilities; clarity about the task; sufficient staff to undertake the job as defined by the expectations of residents, regulators and so of the management itself.

Consideration of *individual staff and residents* leads us to the importance of establishing systems: first, those for the appointing of staff to attract the best and to keep out inappropriate people; second, to support staff; and, third, to observe and think about individual residents, in particular those who may be most vulnerable.

The category, *worker style*, relates to the establishment of a staff team that has its first loyalty to the care of residents and works openly, so challenging the secrecy on which abuse thrives.

Another way of creating a climate in which abuse is made less probable is to consider the circumstances when appropriate boundaries are more likely to be transgressed. Abuse is more likely when:

- a staff member works alone, and there is little oversight and supervision;
- work is in private – away from other residents;
- staff are under pressure;
- people don't know their rights;
- residents are at a low ebb – frightened, tired, depressed or at nighttimes;
- there is discouragement of showing, and talking about, feelings;
- there are no acceptable or easy ways for staff to talk about their concerns in their own work or those of others;
- there is no clarity that the overriding loyalty is to the task and the residents, *not* to one's colleagues.

Types of abuse or bad practice

Managers and regulators need knowledge of what may go wrong; they need also to be alert to different types of abuse. These have been categorised as:

- institutionalised practices;

- indifference and neglect;
- physical cruelty;
- humiliation;
- too authoritarian a life-style;
- a dull and depressing life-style;
- an overcrowded and run down environment;
- disharmony amongst the staff team;
- staff misappropriating goods or money;
- residents' abuse of residents and of staff;
- an improper influence on the life-style of others; and
- sexual abuse.

(Clough 1999a)

Such knowledge should be used to lead those with responsibility to check what is happening against the clues as to what may go wrong.

Interpretation of information

When inquiries review abusive events and causation, one of the stark findings is that frequently concerns about the home have been raised earlier, often by more than one person. The people who expressed those concerns most often were staff, but were also relatives, other visitors such as students and, at times, residents. For example, one resident 'went to the Town Hall and said that he wanted to leave Nye Bevan Lodge because it was like a concentration camp (he had been in one during the war)' (Gibbs *et al.* 1987: 27).

Complaints like this may have been examined and discarded, examined and acted on (but ineffectually) or ignored. So, one of the key lessons, cited in literature on abuse of children, is that concerns have to be taken seriously. Sometimes the expression of anxiety will turn out to be a misinterpretation of events. On other occasions, an event may turn out to be a single episode, out of character with the individual or the place; this is not satisfactory but differs from a situation where the individual event is an indication of practices that are repeated on other occasions or with other residents. However, there may be substance to the allegation.

Thus, we move into one of the key areas for management and regulators: how is the individual event to be interpreted?

There are many competing interests. Staff and their unions properly do not want guilt assumed before an investigation has taken place; nor do they want records kept when staff were not found guilty of the offence. Management often argues to regulators that people who make complaints, particularly former staff, may have a grudge. This may be true, yet the information given may also be true. Importantly, staff may also make mistakes, perhaps in errors of judgement as to residents' ability to manage to bath themselves or, on a stressful day, losing their temper with a resident who is being unkind to someone else. It is imperative that there is capacity and space to interpret the individual event.

One way to do this is to look for any evidence of a pattern. Once again, a study of inquiry reports shows that frequently, in retrospect, a pattern can be seen. The task for managers and regulators is to search for patterns at an early stage. A single event is to be seen in a wider context: is there any other evidence that raises anxieties?

The focus of such attention could be on the well-being of a particular resident: is there any evidence of bruising, frequency of falls, appearing fearful of some or all staff or residents, depression? Alternatively, a particular member of staff or staff members could be considered: have there been other complaints, substantiated or not?; how do they manage their task? do they appear to be out of control, drinking alcohol or reporting sick frequently? Another area to examine could be particular times of the day: this may indicate stressful work patterns at certain times, for example arrangements perceived as problematic for meals or bathing; or there may be occasions when staff work more privately or when a resident has more opportunity, unnoticed, to assault another.

Given the importance of patterns, it is essential that records are kept of occasions when staff have been investigated and no evidence has been found of wrongdoing. Personnel practice may demand destruction of such information, but this would inhibit the ability of managers or, more likely, regulators to become alert that a particular complaint is one of several similar comments that have been made. Somehow, procedures have to be found that will protect staff but allow for such records to be kept, though not as part of individual staff files.

Prevalence indicators

It is worthwhile for managers and regulators to try to place an individual event in context. There are other *predisposing factors* that could act like alarm bells (Clough 1999a). The first is whether or not there have been previous complaints and, if so, their number, time-scale and the numbers of staff involved. A second factor is the state of the buildings; an establishment that appears run down may be an indication of a lack of interest in what happens.

A third predisposing factor is staffing problems: frequency of shortages and sickness; high turnover; little supervision, in particular at night; high consumption of alcohol; poor attitude and behaviour towards residents; and discord amongst the staff team. Given the significance of senior staff to the life of a home, it is not surprising that their failure to function well is a fourth indicator of potential problems shown in absence, lack of interest, preoccupation with events in their own lives and being in post for a very long time.

The fifth factor is found in resident characteristics: those with few visitors, who rarely go out or are regarded as highly demanding, awkward or problematic are more likely to be abused. An indicator of a potential problem is the demeanour and response of residents to staff. Finally, long-standing uncertainty about the future of the establishment does seem to lead to loss of morale.

Action/inaction

The reasons for staff and managers' failing to take early action lie partly in not knowing what seriousness to attach to the information available at a particular time. However, there are additional factors. Lack of agreement about purpose and task may lead to uncertainty about what should be happening. Inadequate resources, whether of buildings or staff, may result in low morale and feelings of the work always being out of control. Frequently, there is confusion and lack of knowledge about guidelines, both amongst staff and residents. The appointment of unsuitable staff or lack of training may lead to unquestioning acceptance. Sadly, the low status ascribed to the work may result in people not being very bothered about what happens in the home, particularly when coupled with anxieties as to where someone might move if they are to move from the home.

Perhaps the most important task for regulators is to create a climate in which their work is recognised as being significant for the well-being of potentially vulnerable residents. Regulation should not be seen as going through the motions.

The first task for regulators is to create an environment in which they model good practice, for example by working as openly as possible with all interested parties, avoiding alliances with any one group, listening to people and taking complaints seriously. They have to make themselves known to anyone with an interest in the home and be available to receive comments about practice.

Second, it is essential that regulators are clear as to the primary task of the home and make judgements about practice against the primary task. A third critical factor is to be clear as to their own role, and able to distinguish between when they are giving advice and making demands. As a part of this function they should observe for themselves, examining the systems in place in the home, in relation to staffing and care; this is followed by making their own judgements. Finally, they have to be prepared to take action.

Secrecy

Sometimes outsiders are surprised that residents keep things to themselves. This surprise fails to understand the pressures for secrecy. People may be frightened of what will happen to them if they talk. They may be ashamed of talking about events, feeling contaminated by the things that have happened. There may be pragmatic reasons for doing nothing: they may think that they will not be believed; they may not know that what has been done to them was wrong or illegal; they may not know their rights; and they may think that nobody will do anything, and therefore that the energy given to exposing the abuse is not worthwhile (of course, they may know that on previous occasions an organisation has taken no action).

Finally, they may have misplaced loyalty to people or the place where the abuse occurs, perhaps being persuaded that the interests of others means that they should not relate what has happened to them.

Thus, there are a number of reasons for not telling anyone about what has happened. However, the notion of 'keeping a secret' introduces forces that, more actively, endeavour to keep matters untold than does the earlier statement of not telling. The 'keeping of secrets' establishes a bond between all of those who know of the event and say nothing to others. The notion of secrecy differs from that of confidentiality: confidentiality is about treating with respect information about others that may be of an intimate nature; and it includes ideas of trust (the 'confidence' of confidentiality). The trust relates to the expectation that the knowledge imparted will be treated properly. Alternatively, the bond in secrecy is based on collective 'not telling', where there is no aspect of dealing appropriately with the information.

Different groups of people may keep quiet for different reasons:

1   *Residents*: because of vulnerability and dependence, despair and feelings that nobody listens; not knowing their rights; fear derived from threats; shame; ambivalence towards the abuser; or thinking that they will be blamed.

2 *Relatives*: because of fear for the well-being of the resident; not believing the resident; or having no other place for the resident to go.

3 *Staff*: because of misplaced loyalty; not knowing when or how to tell others ('to blow the whistle'); their own involvement (implicit or explicit) in the event; or fear of other staff.

4 *Managers*: because matters are kept from them; they may not bother or know how to find out what is going on; fear of an individual, in particular the internal manager if he or she is a powerful personality; fear of tackling people on bad practice; or not knowing how the organisation will cope if the place closes.

5 *People*: as insiders may keep matters secret from outsiders.

Openness

Staff who talk with certainty and apparent knowledge may set themselves up and be seen by others as experts in the field. Once there is even local recognition of someone's competence or expertise, it may be difficult for others to raise questions about their practice. In particular, some establishments (and the people who manage them) have become recognised as willing to take in as residents people who are hard to place, indeed those whom other places reject. The combination of being willing to take troubled and troublesome people *and* of being recognised as having expertise is powerful (see Stanley's discussion of Beck in Chapter 1 of this volume).

Kennard advocates the creation of an open environment. Specifically he has advice for staff: 'Look on this as an opportunity to learn about yourself as well as others'; 'Get involved with what is going on'; and 'Be yourself … say what you actually feel. … Don't hold back for fear of saying the wrong thing' (1983: 126). In the end it is the spirit of openness and questioning that drives out secrecy. The responsibility to create this rests on everyone. But it rests particularly strongly on those with formal responsibility for the activity of residential and nursing-home care. A climate has to be created in which there is an expectation that people will talk about life and work in the home. Managers, internal and external, and regulators must work in a way that models the life-style they want to see created; they must be straightforward in their negotiations and open to questions from others about the way they work. The consequence will be that staff, relatives and residents will know that thinking, enquiring and discussing are life enhancing activities.

222   *Roger Clough*

References

Burton, J. (1998) *Managing Residential Care*, London: Routledge.

Clough, R. (1988) 'Scandals in residential care', unpublished paper commissioned by the Wagner Committee.

—— (ed.) (1994) *Insights into Inspection: The Regulation of Social Care*, London: Whiting & Birch.

—— (ed.) (1996) *The Abuse of Care in Residential Institutions*, London: Whiting & Birch.

—— (1999a) 'Scandalous care: Interpreting public enquiry reports of scandals in residential care', *Journal of Elder Abuse and Neglect* 10(1/2) (forthcoming).

—— (1999b) *Practising Residential Work*, Basingstoke: Macmillan (forthcoming).

Department of Health and Social Security and Welsh Office (1973) *Local Authority Building Note 2 – Guidelines for Residential Accommodation for Elderly People*, London: HMSO.

Gibbs, J., Evans, M. and Rodway, S. (1987) *Report of the Inquiry into Nye Bevan Lodge*, London: London Borough of Southwark Social Services Department.

Goldsmith, M. (1997) 'Hearing their voice', in S. Hunter (ed.) (1997) *Dementia: Challenges and New Directions*, London: Jessica Kingsley.

Kennard, D. (1983) *An Introduction to Therapeutic Communities*, London: Routledge and Kegan Paul.

King, R., Raynes, N. and Tizard, J. (1971) *Patterns of Residential Care*, London: Routledge and Kegan Paul.

Parker, R. (1988) 'Children', in I. Sinclair (ed.) (1988) *Residential Care: The Research Reviewed*, London: HMSO.

Residential Forum (1997) *Managing a Home from Home*, London: Residential Forum.

Rowlings, C. (1995) 'Elder abuse in context', in R. Clough (ed.) *Elder Abuse and the Law*, London: Action on Elder Abuse.

11 Conclusion

Shifting the focus, from 'bad apples' to users' rights

Jill Manthorpe and Nicky Stanley

The approach taken in this volume has allowed us to bring together a range of different voices and analyses that have described and deconstructed institutional abuse. Some common themes have emerged across a number of chapters. There are also some significant differences in the ways in which abuse is constructed and experienced by distinct user groups, as well as in the ways in which the State and the public conceptualise institutional abuse in relation to these groups. Different values and expectations surround the care of children, adults with learning disabilities, adults with mental health problems and older people. This conclusion aims to identify some of these differences as well as focusing on similarities. In attempting to find answers to the questions posed by institutional abuse the differences may be as illuminating as the similarities. Whilst some of the prevention and response strategies considered here are appropriate for all groups across the life course, others may have relevance for one group only. In seeking to develop our analysis, we have tried to avoid reductive simplifications and to maintain a view that is multifaceted yet comprehensible.

Inquiries and public perceptions

It is clear from a reading of this book that much of the evidence concerning institutional abuse in the United Kingdom derives from inquiry reports. This is in part a consequence of the fact that research into experience of abuse is difficult to design and implement, and easy to criticise on methodological grounds. However, the tradition of the public inquiry in the United Kingdom has become well-established in the late twentieth century and inquiries and the ensuing public interest have become powerful levers in the creation of social policy. Reder and Duncan (1996) have identified the purposes of inquiries as discipline, learning, catharsis and reassurance, and they note that these agendas can often conflict. These processes can also be enacted at different levels so that both policy makers and individual practitioners can learn from the lessons of inquiries, and catharsis can be experienced by individual victims as well as by the general public. Learning and reassurance tend to be the predominant themes in the inquiry reports considered in this volume. Prior to the establishment of the North Wales Tribunal in 1997, concerns were expressed by the local authority's insurers that publication of an inquiry report could result in a flood of compensation claims (Elias 1997) and liability is now an issue that could be added to Reder and Duncan's list.

Children's institutions have attracted the greatest number of public inquiries. This is more likely to be an indication of the nature of the public response to disclosure of abuse of children in institutional care than it is to reflect the incidence of abuse. Failures to protect children in residential care evoke a particularly strong response because many of the children in such institutions have been placed there as a result of State intervention in family life. British social legislation continues to betray unease about such intervention (Fox-Harding 1991) and abuse of children who are 'looked after' by the State may be seen to undermine the State's claim to intervene to protect.

By contrast, older people, or at least their families, are considered to be exercising choice when they enter institutional care. The language and transactions of the commercial world have penetrated the residential care sector for older people to such an extent that care has come to be conceptualised as a commodity that is bought, if not by the consumer directly, by the State on behalf of the consumer. Abuse constitutes a failure to meet a contract of care but does not have the wider implications for Government policy that can be identified in the case of children who experience institutional abuse.

Users of mental health services are currently least likely to find their experiences the subject of public inquiries. The only cases of abuse in mental health institutions that have attracted significant levels of public interest in recent years are those that have occurred in the high-profile special hospitals (see Blom-Cooper 1992 and Prins *et al.* 1993). Elsewhere, as Jennie Williams and Frank Keating argue in Chapter 6, the low status ascribed to mental health service users and the readiness to label complaints as pathology means that allegations of abuse are rarely brought to public attention.

Adults with learning disabilities share the label of deviancy attributed to those with mental health problems but, as both chapters covering adults with learning disabilities note, they are often infantilised and associated with the innocence of childhood. The contrasted labels of innocence or deviancy are predominant in the discourse surrounding different groups and their experience of institutional abuse. As Chapter 1 argues, in the case of children in residential care, there is much confusion as to whether they are innocent children who require protection or disturbed and sexually active adolescents. Colton and Vanstone's (1996) collection of the personal accounts of those who abuse such children offers evidence of a similar emphasis on the deviant or 'spoilt' identity of the child in the thinking and the minimisation strategies of abusers.

A new approach to conceptualising the position of those in institutional care would identify them as signatories to a contract of care that conferred a right to protection. The image of older people in residential and nursing care as consumers is a move towards this position but, at present, their rights as consumers are extremely limited. The labels of innocence and deviance serve only to objectify those receiving institutional care and render them vulnerable to abuse. The focus on users' voices in this volume allows us to shift those who live in institutions to the centre-stage and to identify them as subjects with complex experiences that resist labelling.

Accountability

A number of the chapters in this book (see those by Nicky Stanley, Christine Barter and Hilary Brown) have identified the recent focus on paedophiles as an unhelpful shift to the 'bad apple' model, which locates institutional abuse in the deviant individual and thereby draws attention away from the wider contexts of the institutional regime and the social structures that shape life in the institution. This focus derives less from inquiry reports that, in meeting their discipline function, tend to examine structures for accountability at a number of levels, but rather from Government statements and media reports.

Such statements tend to emphasise the 'cleverness' and 'cunning' of individual abusers who 'infiltrate' or 'penetrate' institutions (see Utting 1997) in order to abuse residents. Language of this sort (in addition to carrying obvious connotations of male sexuality) conveys the idea that abusers come into institutions from the world outside. The abuser is thus disassociated from the institution. His 'cleverness' and ability to hoodwink others signals the helplessness of the organisation in the face of the threat posed by such individuals.

The stated intention underlying this picture of the individual abuser is to alert both those working in, and managing, institutions and the general public. However, a sense of panic is also discernible here and can be traced to those reports that associate individual abusers with settings that were once considered 'safe' and respectable. The two most prominent examples of such settings are the Church and independent boarding schools. The Roman Catholic Church has been particularly damaged by reports of institutional abuse in children's homes and residential schools that it managed in the North West of England and, when taken together with other reports of child abuse involving both the Church in Ireland (Moore 1995) and the Anglican Church (Davies 1998), the churches' image as offering a place of safe refuge has been badly damaged. Similarly, the conviction of Dennis Grain on charges of sexual abuse in 1995 had the effect of drawing Eton College, one of the most prestigious independent boarding schools in the UK (where he had worked for a year as a housemaster), into the sphere of institutions that have harboured paedophiles (Connett and Calvert 1997).

An emphasis on individual abusers evokes the danger of concentrating resources and energy on issues of detection rather than examining the internal regimes of institutions and the ways in which they may feed or shelter abusive dynamics. The image of the pathologised paedophile penetrating the sanctity of the institution reinforces the application of objectifying labels of innocence and deviance to those living in institutions as discussed above. While effective filters need to be in place to ensure that the appointment of staff is as informed a process as possible, a focus on the individual abuser may serve to deflect attention from the organisation and culture of institutions, from social attitudes towards the task and recipients of care, and from the experience of users.

Whistle-blowing

The history of abuse within institutions is also a history of whistle-blowing within UK welfare services. Whistle-blowers' accounts of practices or incidents have provided the impetus for a number of high-profile inquiries from that of Ely Hospital to the North Wales Tribunal. While Vernon may argue that it has been transformed from a 'vice to a virtue' (1998: 222) it remains the case that to act as a whistle-blower both challenges individual security and relationships, and serves to identify only certain forms of abuse. It is only staff who function within institutions as whistle-blowers and transgress the boundary with the outside world. Framed as complainants or witnesses, residents are not seen to possess the inside status, expertise or professionalism of staff. What staff identify through whistle-blowing is their subjective and professional views of the actions of their peers or managers.

One key area related to whistle-blowing is the protection necessary to avoid recriminations, though in many cases relationships may have already reached a low ebb or employment may have ceased. Alison Taylor, former Director of Social Services in Gwynedd, identifies her whistle-blowing as 'professional suicide', for she was suspended from her senior post in social services on the grounds that she 'had fabricated allegations of abuse and that this caused a breakdown in professional relationships' (1998: 60). While there are calls for whistle-blowing charters in respect of both public and private spheres of employment, Taylor's account presents a picture of current cultural norms within organisations. Calls for legislative reform may promote organisational openness but seem unlikely to transform the highly charged emotional atmosphere when an 'insider' breaks organisational codes of loyalty and self-preservation.

Institutional care in its various forms seems to create settings where an introspective culture is viewed as both acceptable and functional. Staff working in such groupings may be encouraged to develop a subset of loyalties to the home or unit and these are fostered by socialisation and the blurring of work and social boundaries. In creating a 'homely' home for residents, staff may become emotionally attached to the staff and resident group and invest themselves heavily in the institution's operations and future. The commercial sector of care may take such self-identification further by tying up individuals' livelihoods and reputations in commercial definitions of success but, as a number of inquiries and scandals mentioned above have demonstrated, a shared value base, for example, in religion may also provide an ethical framework in which abuses can be ignored or invalidated.

The debate about whistle-blowing needs to be extended to other forms of reporting and in particular the willingness and ability of organisations to respond to anonymous allegations. Anonymity, like whistle-blowing, may be perceived as a status that negates the value of the message. Very clear messages from inspecting and regulatory bodies need to be given concerning their willingness to consider anonymous reporting. Survivors' organisations and self-help groups may also face dilemmas in this area when they are given information in the expectation that it will be kept confidential. ChildLine's experiences in this area, as described by Mary MacLeod in Chapter 2, may be useful to others seeking to assist members or those making enquiries.

Whistle-blowing has also another characteristic: it is highly subjective. It appears to be only worth the risk if the abuse or neglect is judged so blatant that an individual feels it worth paying the price (however calculated). The initial motivation for raising issues may be located in a transgression of the individual's professional or personal values. Thus, abuses may have to be stark or sizeable. The survey reported by Hunt and Campbell (1998) of social workers, despite its low response rate, found that serious incidents of abuse such as physical, sexual or financial abuse were clearly identified as matters that had to be reported. Other areas of misconduct such as verbal abuse were not so clear and a more 'flexible' interpretation was placed on them.

A number of chapters in this book allude to the issue of degrees of abuse and this is clearly one area in which the language of abuse has been unhelpful. There are without doubt differences in degree or severity, and labelling poor practice as abuse may create a climate of fear for those considering residential care and stigmatise those associated with it through their experience as users or as workers in the system. Both the social work and nursing professions have suffered from their associations with poor-quality services. A culture that elevates whistle-blowing may also dissolve the relationships of trust and reliance that characterise a job where teamwork and round-the-clock continuity of care is essential.

Whistle-blowing therefore may be only one way forward in developing staff's ability to bring matters of concern to the attention of the public or commissioners of services. As a conduit for messages that have been deliberately suppressed by the managerial equivalent of 'bad apple practitioners' whistle-blowing may be the best approach, but it should be a last resort.

Far less commonly encountered in the practice literature or policy guidance are alternatives to whistle-blowing for staff. Much has been made of the complaints business within social and health care but this is generally applied to service users. As the accounts in the chapters by Les Bright, and Jeanette Copperman and Julie McNamara point out, complaints mechanisms do not always meet the needs of service users. However, they exist and to some extent are appropriate. A publication such as this does not identify their positive outcomes. Similar mechanisms are not available for staff and their own responses to complaints can become defensive as they seek to ensure the continuity of contracts or maintain the organisation's reputation.

For professionals, the ability to draw on their codes of conduct and professional status provides some counterweight to the business or contract culture of care. However, as most staff within residential settings are not professionally qualified this defence is not available. New moral imperatives have to be created around care: a task that is difficult to do among a demoralised, often part-time and transient staff group. In many ways whistle-blowing is attractive because of its position in clear moral territory: the David versus the Goliath with a clear sense of what is right and wrong. Training staff in how to whistle-blow may not be the most comprehensive way of improving care standards overall, and other ways of empowering staff need to be found that recognise their dilemmas but also their desires to improve matters incrementally rather than 'explode' issues and their organisational or professional concerns.

Regulation

The risks of employing those who are termed 'inappropriate people' in caring professions (see, for example, the discussion paper by two Directors of Social Services, Boyle and Leadbetter 1998) can be addressed by a variety of approaches. Interestingly, the purpose and value of police checks are subject to substantial critique whilst simultaneously it is argued that they should be extended to those working with vulnerable adults as well as children. Boyle and Leadbetter raise the point that the meaning of previous convictions has to be established and a decision made about the weight that will be given to the offence. Our experience as admissions officers for a qualifying social-work programme has given us cause for concern about the potential for discretion in relation to declared offences. Highly subjective decisions are taken in relation to the type of offence, age at conviction, the applicant's own account and the attitudes of managers within local partner agencies. Such an approach may result in an informed risk assessment but the absence of consensus about such a framework may mean that practice is highly variable.

This picture of patchy scrutiny extends to the more troubled issues of suspicion and concerns. As Boyle and Leadbetter point out, there is no central database for people who have been classed as 'unfit' to operate residential care services (1998: 14). The position over exchanging information between agencies is also unclear. However, unproven allegations or mere suspicions are not 'hard' information and need to be balanced with civil rights and fair employment practices. Nicky Stanley's chapter in his book identifies residential childcare workers' anxiety in the face of their vulnerability to allegations of abuse. Van Heeswyk (1998) highlights the importance for support and supervision at individual and group level, to work on staff's feelings of ambivalence and uncertainty in this area.

Staff supervision is more developed, however, in some areas of residential social care than in others. Indeed, the meaning of supervision may be interpreted differently within institutions that follow different models or owe their organisational pattern to one discipline or sector. Few institutions, generally only those 'in trouble', utilise outside consultants to offer supervision to the group, managers or individual staff. As Webb and McCaffrey (1998) illustrate, even consultants can find it difficult to work with staff once an event such as exposure of a staff member as a possible abuser has happened and, as Christine Barter argues in Chapter 3, we need to develop systems for responding to such events in ways that can be positive.

Much will be expected from legislation following the White Paper *Modernising Social Services* (Department of Health 1998), in which the extent of policy concern about standards of care in institutions is clearly evident. The introduction of a General Social Care Council, for example, is set in a context of a largely unqualified and untrained workforce (80 per cent), of no national mechanism to establish and enforce standards of care and conduct, and a lack of confidence in existing education and training in the area. The drawing up of codes of conduct will be one of the first priorities of the Council: a code of conduct for individual staff and a code of practice for employers. However, the White Paper envisages a narrower registration framework than the broad sweep of the Council's name might suggest, limiting it to qualified social workers and residential childcare workers who have gained NVQ Level 3. The heads of adult care homes will be 'appropriately qualified' and they too might be a group that it would be 'helpful' to register (1998: 5.23); the Government, however, continues to identify with the view that residential childcare is qualitatively different. As many of the chapters in this book demonstrate, there is now much in common between institutions providing services across the life course and issues of control and choice are not confined to one age group.

The White Paper also announces a new independent watch-dog for care homes and other provision. With the proposed name of Commissions for Care Standards, these eight regional bodies are to have 'tough new powers' to counter existing practice and policies. The White Paper identifies problems with lack of independence, lack of coherence and lack of consistency in the current regulatory system and intends to counter this with the establishment of such commissions, independent statutory bodies but with strong central control from the Department of Health (1998: 4.7). It is clear that centralisation is one major theme of this White Paper both in strengthening the overall inspection role of the Department but also in setting up national frameworks for the training and activities of inspectors.

A series of extensions to existing inspectorate activities are proposed by the White Paper, such as the bringing into one system the variety of approaches to children's homes and the introduction of inspection for small private children's homes (1998: 4.35). Additionally, a Children's Rights Officer will be appointed for each Commission for Care Standards. The thinking behind this appears to be that such a post will ensure children's welfare is 'not swamped by the much larger volume of adult services that the Commission will deal with' (1998: 4.41). This approach will have to be monitored, for there is a danger that such a post and emphasis will again reinforce the idea that residential work with children is in some way more testing for staff. As we have illustrated, this view may not necessarily be correct and again may lead to differences in the assessment and management of risk. What is to be welcomed, however, is the term Rights Officer, for it points to a recognition that it is a resident's or service user's right not to be abused in institutional care. All age groups, however, should have the language of rights extended to their care, for rights are generally more enforceable than statements about quality or need.

The White Paper is more firmly grounded in the residential child-care sector than in the broader institutional-care framework. The position of psychiatric patients is, of course, excluded from the White Paper as responsibility for their care falls to health providers in the main and their separate systems of inspection and accountability. However, many mental health services are now provided by agencies falling under the social care umbrella. The White Paper's focus is predominantly on children and older people's services and it will be important, as it moves on to the legislative calendar, for mental health residential services to ensure that their needs are met by the new systems. As the chapters by Copperman and McNamara and by Williams and Keating indicate, far less is known about mental health residential services other than psychiatric hospital provision. In comparison with Frank Glendenning's discussion of elder abuse, work on abuse in mental health settings in the UK has been little informed by international developments.

Roger Clough's chapter serves as a reminder that regulation and inspection systems operate at many levels. If the new commissions are to concentrate on their 'policing' role rather than operating as agencies which attempt to work with providers to raise standards, then this function will have to be developed elsewhere. Hard decisions will still have to be made about organisations or institutions that are borderline rather than overtly inadequate or run by evident abusers. Inspection and registration may assist in identifying abusers but reaching a decision about the point where an institution provides inadequate care will remain a complex process. New guidance or codes of practice will have to be developed to support the inspectorates and it will be helpful if these include assistance with decision making: one key system that is often left under-developed.

Training

Training is one of the central themes of the White Paper. The stated aim of improving the qualification levels of all those engaged in social care includes among its first objectives the achievement of NVQ Level 3 for all residential childcare workers and qualification at Diploma in Social Work (DipSW) level for all heads of homes (those in residential childcare having already benefited from the Residential Child Care Initiative). A more qualified workforce is likely to be a more stable workforce, and therefore more easily monitored as well as offering increased skills. Furthermore, higher levels of training across all groups of staff should make for a more critical and questioning workforce that is less likely to be impressed by the pseudo-therapy of a Frank Beck figure. However, there is nothing in the White Paper to suggest that new qualification structures are being contemplated. The social pedagogue model for childcare advocated by Warner in 1992 and, more recently in Scotland, by Kent (1997) appears to have been put back on the shelf by the Government.

The continued reliance on existing models for training will ensure that the National Vocational Qualification (NVQ) structure will remain the most widespread form of accreditation available to those working in residential care settings. NVQ awards are aimed less at changing practice and more at the identification and valuing of skills and knowledge that are already owned. This reduces their effectiveness as a tool for challenging and transforming abusive practice. While the Government has initiated a review of the content of Diploma in Social Work programmes, questions remain about the status of residential care within such programmes.

Training that aims to tackle abuse in institutional settings needs to move beyond the issue of identifying abuse to examine questions of what constitutes an effective response to abuse once it has been identified. As Les Bright notes in his chapter, participants on training courses do not find it difficult to identify abusive or unacceptable practice. While organisations may provide procedures and guidance to cover gross abuse such as sexual abuse, a number of contributors to this book have noted the difficulty of challenging behaviour that falls into the category of emotional abuse. Training aimed at combating abuse should incorporate users' perspectives and, ideally, involve users themselves in the delivery of training. As this book should have demonstrated, users' voices serve to break down the distancing and labelling mechanisms that objectify the experience of abuse.

Gender and patriarchy

The introduction to this book identified gender as offering a useful perspective to understanding the world of institutions and the dynamics of abuse. This theme is explored in a number of chapters (see those by Nicky Stanley, Hilary Brown and Jennie Williams and Frank Keating). The life course approach makes it possible to distinguish the differences in institutional patterns, noting, for example, the highly problematic area of men being involved in intimate care tasks or in close proximity to vulnerable children or adults and the way this is constructed as transgressing sexual boundaries. Just as the abuse of people with learning disabilities is dominated by concerns about sexual vulnerability, so issues around gender focus on sexual behaviour. This serves to draw attention away from other forms of abuse and to construct problems about men's and women's places in the delivery of care.

New thinking in this area may help to identify some of the commonalities of experience between those who work in and those who live in residential services. The low status of female care assistants in residential and nursing care for older people, for example, may resonate with the low status in old age of residents. Both may be unwilling occupants of the institution.

Thompson *et al.* draw attention to the position of women working within learning disability services seeking to protect themselves from abuse. Their study indicates that female staff are 'differentially subjected' (1997: 580) to men's abusive behaviour, recording a ratio of eighteen women to one man subjected to such behaviour. In their view, female staff were caught between the pressures to be caring and yet professional. They had to make 'isolated, individual responses' (1997: 574) to sexualised behaviour and could not rely on supervisors or managers to set and sustain legitimate role boundaries.

In some respects, the solution to such problems can be seen as the withdrawal of women from providing intimate care for male residents. Thompson *et al.*, pointing to the problem for female staff when residents sought physical contact or embarrassing proximity, identify proposed solutions as including more male staff in personal care, such as bathing. Others might find this approach fraught with hazards. A seemingly simple solution such as male-provided intimate care may decrease the likelihood of risk to female staff but increase other risks. The perspectives of staff engaged in intimate or personal care may serve to unpick the association between 'victim' and resident if such staff feel abused and relatively powerless to complain or to draw attention to their embarrassment and discomfort.

It is perhaps too narrow a perspective to confine gender to issues of sexuality. A life course approach offers a broader focus on issues of power and one theme that emerges is the gendered nature of the hierarchy within institutions. While the majority of care and domestic staff are women, the role of the institutional head or manager is often held by a man. Such a replication of patterns of patriarchy with a father figure as the head of the household can help explain some of the dynamics of institutional life. Homes or units that use the image of a 'family' to convey a sense of their closeness and security may reinforce this sense of paternal patterning of relationships. The position of male heads of units or institutions with women as their deputies or staff may evoke feelings of untrammelled authority and dependency. In such an atmosphere, the barriers to challenging practices or policy can feel insurmountable.

Attention to the nature and sources of managerial power may identify other dynamics that inform or support abusive practices. While the terms superintendent or officer-in-charge may be less commonly encountered nowadays, the militaristic patterns of control associated with these designations may linger on and impinge on the lives of staff as well as residents. The expansion of private and voluntary sector provision where ownership and management may be 'family businesses' or cottage industries (Wistow 1995) places particular strain on professional and personal boundaries, and contributes to a blurring between them.

In such settings, particularly those run by husband and wife teams, patterns of power in families are particularly likely to be reproduced and the position of staff who are not involved in ownership of the business may be especially weak. As the Office of Fair Trading report (1998) notes, most providers of residential homes are independent small businesses with one or two homes, while the very small homes tend to specialise in care for younger people with physical or multiple disabilities. Consequently, the very small home (under four residents) may well have family-like characteristics with younger people receiving care and older staff or owner/managers 'in charge'. As the chapters on learning disabilities and older people illustrate, age is a variable that is rarely considered in the dynamics of inter-personal relationships within residential care, and further research would be helpful in formulating ideas about the extent to which staff responses are informed by age differentials.

The conceptualisation of adult residents as children may provide much of the context for emotional abuse. Regular humiliation is one aspect of abusive behaviour that is closely linked to issues of control within institutional settings. Chappell reports how residents in the homes for people with learning disabilities she studied were 'under scrutiny' or observation much of their time, and some spoke of 'getting watched' (1994: 429). Associated with this lack of privacy was the way personal information or criticism was made public. She found that people were embarrassed, distressed and had no redress.

Such accounts provide evidence for the devaluing of those in institutional settings and the confusion of public and private in institutional life. We have little evidence about the effects of criticism and negative labelling in terms of precise harm, but further listening and observation may help identify the impact of continual psychological pressure. Attention also needs to be given to the ways in which patterns of gender, ownership and age serve to objectify and infantilise residents while simultaneously creating organisations where male authority cannot be challenged.

Abuse between residents

A key theme in the chapters of this book has been the pervasive nature and damaging effects of abuse between residents of institutions. Such abuse may be the end-product of a 'bullying culture' where interactions between residents contribute to maintaining hierarchies that place the staff firmly at the top of the pecking order. Abusive or controlling behaviour on the part of staff may be mirrored within the resident group and may serve a common function of keeping everyone 'in their place'. Abuse between residents seems most likely where there is limited scope for meeting individual users' needs and little attention has been given to matching or balancing the resident group. Some of the examples of such settings covered in this book are a mix of young abusers and children who have been abused in children's homes, mixed sex psychiatric wards and the use of long-stay residential homes for older people to provide respite care for confused and disinhibited individuals. Many admissions to institutional care occur as emergencies or under crisis conditions and, in such circumstances, consideration of the group's needs and the information required to plan for them is often inadequate.

Just as staff may seek to compensate for their own sense of powerlessness within the organisation by exerting control over users (Wardhaugh and Wilding 1993), so residents, deprived of autonomy and social status, may attempt to affirm their sense of control and power at the expense of other, more vulnerable residents. Such behaviour is not surprising; what matters is the response that it evokes. It is particularly troubling that abuse between residents appears to elicit limited concern from staff with high levels of tolerance extended to behaviour such as sexual assault in psychiatric wards and residential and nursing homes (see Chapters 6 and 9), and recruitment into prostitution among children in residential homes and women on psychiatric wards (see Chapters 1 and 7). The users' accounts included in this book indicate that abuse between residents is under-recorded and frequently connived at by staff. This lack of response reflects low expectations and objectification of those receiving institutional care. This is an area where staff attitudes need to be challenged and significantly modified. Further work might usefully seek to identify the extent to which abuse between users is linked to coercive and abusive care regimes.

Users' voices

While the focus of several of the contributions to this book has been on users' views it is evident from them all that acquiring users' views is a complex process. All chapters point to ways in which users' views are to some extent mediated by those who receive their messages, and one finding that emerges from this book is the involvement of family members in articulating this voice for some users of institutional services but not others. Relationships between residents and their families when residents are elderly or have learning disabilities appear to be sustained in many instances despite the move to residential care and the physical separation. Some relatives appear to be 'part of the scene' and continue to occupy important positions in monitoring quality of care at all levels. They appear sensitive to the possibility of abuse, in all its forms, notably its emotional dimension.

However, in children's homes and in mental health services the views of relatives are less evident. This might at a superficial glance be ascribed to the deviance label applied to residents and the possibility of construing their institutional residence as a matter of shame for the wider family group. Alternatively, staff within such institutions may find it difficult to engage with families effectively, particularly if family dynamics or actions have contributed to entry to an institution. However, we should avoid stereotyping family relationships among different age groups, for many older people in residential care have no living relatives to provide support, or ties may have broken down for them or for other individuals at various stages of the life course. Some models of advocacy services recognise this as an important variable among residents and seek to target their services on those without families, offering befriending or help with personal finances. Such services, however, are scarce and there is no indication in the White Paper, *Modernising Social Services*, that a national system to develop advocacy will supplement the more organisationally focused systems of regulation and inspection.

To some extent, as we have seen in the chapters here, the existence of pressure groups may provide opportunities for relatives to organise around issues of quality or concern in residential services. Following the movement of certain client groups from long-stay health service provision in hospitals to community-based institutions and homes, organised groups of relatives have continued to focus on their members' well-being. In some instances this concern may be inter-preted by staff and indeed by residents as intrusive and risk-averse. In other settings residents may feel that staff and family members collude to deprive them of opportunities for ordinary living and the risks entailed (Manthorpe *et al.* 1997). The views of users provided in this book have emphasised that, while abuse in its most obvious forms is clearly unpalatable, some residents also identify other forms of demeaning treatment as abusive. While emotional or psychological abuse is a category developed in relation to childcare, usually between family members, it is still under-developed in respect of care provided by institutions. As Frank Glendenning illustrates, work from North America is leading the field here in relation to older people, and this work seeks to identify ways in which practice may be improved. It will be interesting to see if this impacts on the training envisaged for care staff in the UK under the new national Training Organisations.

The generally low level of expectations among those who reside in institutions is conveyed by the White Paper, *Modernising Social Services*, and by a number of the chapters here. Les Bright, Jennie Williams and Frank Keating all suggest that residents may be inured to the impoverished environment and quality of life within services. Distress and challenging behaviours exhibited by other residents may exacerbate this attitude of resignation or, as Les Bright illustrates, may provoke a feeling that it is best not to be identified as a complainer.

Such an atmosphere makes for particular difficulty in identifying and naming behaviour as emotional or psychological abuse or neglect. While it is easy to call for further research, this area appears to be important for further work. We would argue that such research should extend beyond definition and identification exercises, important and instructive as these are, but should relate clearly to measurement of extent and severity. Neglect too needs to be conceptualised more broadly, in particular to explore what is meant by an impoverished environment and its relation to poverty, inequalities and class. One of the evident negative comparisons that may be made from taking on a life course perspective on institutions is the comparative neglect of matters related to class and social status. To live in an institution appears to remove this important variable from a person's identity.

Towards a framework for users' rights

This book provides a critical if limited overview of rights within institutions, noting the areas where specific legislation has provided residents with a level of protection, by alerting staff to the penalties of crossing certain boundaries but also pointing to wider social debates about rights and accountability. Children in children's homes are most likely to conceive of themselves as having rights, and their language conveys an at least rhetorical impression of certainty. This appears to have been influenced by wider social circumstances such as the publicity around child abuse cases and the establishment of helplines and other sources of assistance and advocacy. For other age groups, however, the language of rights is less well-developed and may be interpreted more negatively by staff. Even in mental health services, where rights have been enshrined by mental health legislation, the rights awarded to users are few in comparison to the rights that are removed.

We end this book with a call for the debate over the future of institutional care to move towards developing a framework of rights for users. This might be achieved through the use of explicit contracts, which could usefully address issues of quality, accountability and regulation. The life course perspective adopted here has illustrated that many of those receiving institutional care are the object of attitudes that reflect social ambivalence towards institutions. Investing users of institutional care with rights may offer a means of shifting resignation and helplessness in the face of abuse.

References

Blom-Cooper, L. (1992) *The Report of the Committee of Inquiry into Complaints about Ashworth Hospital*, London: HMSO.

Boyle, M. and Leadbetter, M. (1998) *Enough is Enough*, London: Elite Recruitment Specialists.

Chappell, A.L. (1994) 'A question of friendship: Community care and the relationships of people with learning difficulties', *Disability and Society* 9(4): 419–34.

Colton, M. and Vanstone, M. (1996) *Betrayal of Trust: Sexual Abuse by Men who Work with Children*, London: Free Association Books.

Connett, D. and Calvert, J. (1997) 'The school for child sex abuse', *Observer*, 9 March, 8–9.

Davies, N. (1998) 'The most secret crime – is the Church forgiving sin or just turning a blind eye?', *Guardian*, 4 June, 6–7.

Department of Health (1998) *Modernising Social Services: Promoting Independence, Improving Protection, Raising Standards*, London: The Stationery Office.

Elias, G. (1997) 'Opening address to the North Wales Tribunal', 21 January 1997, *North Wales Tribunal Transcripts*, Wales.

Fox-Harding, L. (1991) *Perspectives in Child Care Policy*, London: Longman.

Hunt, G. and Campbell, D. (1998) 'Social workers speak out', in G. Hunt (ed.) *Whistleblowing in the Social Services*, London: Arnold.

Kent, R. (1997) *Children's Safeguard Review*, Edinburgh: The Scottish Office.

Manthorpe, J., Walsh, M., Alaszewski, A. and Harrison, L. (1997) 'Issues of risk, practice and welfare in learning disability services', *Disability and Society* 12: 69–82.

Moore, C. (1995) *Betrayal of Trust – The Father Brendan Smyth Affair and the Catholic Church*, Dublin: Marino.

Office of Fair Trading (1998) *Older People as Consumers in Care Homes*, London: Office of Fair Trading.

Prins, H., Backer-Holst, T., Francis, E. and Keitch, I. (1993) *Report of the Committee of Inquiry into the Death at Broadmoor Hospital of Orville Blackwood and a Review of the Deaths of Two Other Afro-Caribbean Patients: Big, Black and Dangerous?*, London: HMSO.

Reder, P. and Duncan, S. (1996) 'Reflections on child abuse inquiries', in J. Peay (ed.) *Inquiries After Homicide*, London: Duckworth.

Taylor, A. (1998) 'Hostages to fortune: The abuse of children in care', in G. Hunt (ed.) *Whistleblowing in the Social Services*, London: Arnold.

Thomson, D., Clare, I. and Brown, H. (1997) 'Not such an "ordinary" relationship: The role of women support staff in relation to men with learning disabilities who have difficult sexual behaviours', *Disability and Society* 12(4): 573–92.

Utting, Sir W. (1997) *People Like Us: The Report of the Review of the Safeguards for Children Living Away from Home*, London: The Stationery Office.

Van Heeswyk, P. (1998) 'In the place of parents: Stress in residential social work with children and adolescents', in R. Davies (ed.) *Stress in Social Work*, London: Jessica Kingsley.

Vernon, S. (1998) 'Legal aspects of whistleblowing in the social services', in G. Hunt (ed.) *Whistleblowing in the Social Services*, London: Arnold.

Wardhaugh, J. and Wilding, P. (1993) 'Towards an explanation of the corruption of care', *Critical Social Policy* 37: 4–31.

Warner, N. (1992) *Choosing with Care: The Report of the Committee of Inquiry into the Selection, Development and Management of Staff in Children's Homes*, London: HMSO.

Webb, L. and McCaffrey, T. (1998) 'Emotional repair for organisations: Intervening in the aftermath of trauma', in R. Davies (ed.) *Stress in Social Work*, London: Jessica Kingsley.

Wistow, G. (1995) 'Aspirations and realities: Community care at the crossroads', *Journal of Health and Social Care in the Community* 3(4): 227–40.

Index